Pediatric Orthopedics

Editor

PATRICK PARENZIN

PHYSICIAN ASSISTANT CLINICS

www.physicianassistant.theclinics.com

Consulting Editor
JAMES A. VAN RHEE

October 2020 • Volume 5 • Number 4

ELSEVIER

1600 John F. Kennedy Boulevard • Suite 1800 • Philadelphia, Pennsylvania, 19103-2899

http://www.theclinics.com

PHYSICIAN ASSISTANT CLINICS Volume 5, Number 4
October 2020 ISSN 2405-7991, ISBN-13: 978-0-323-73393-9

Editor: Katerina Heidhausen
Developmental Editor: Nicholas Henderson

Physician Assistant Clinics (ISSN: 2405–7991) is published quarterly by Elsevier Inc., 360 Park Avenue South, New York, NY 10010-1710. Months of issue are January, April, July, and October. Periodicals postage paid at New York, NY and additional mailing offices. Subscription prices are $150.00 per year (US individuals), $216.00 (US institutions), $100.00 (US students), $150.00 (Canadian individuals), $271.00 (Canadian institutions), $100.00 (Canadian students), $150.00 (international individuals), $271.00 (international institutions), and $100.00 (international students). Foreign air speed delivery is included in all *Clinics* subscription prices. All prices are subject to change without notice. POSTMASTER: Send address changes to *Physician Assistant Clinics*, Elsevier Periodicals Customer Service, 11830 Westline Industrial Drive, St. Louis, MO 63146. Customer Service Health Sciences Division, Subscription Customer Service, 3251 Riverport Lane, Maryland Heights, MO 63043. **Customer Service: 1-800-654-2452 (U.S. and Canada); 314-447-8871 (outside U.S. and Canada). Fax: 314-447-8029. E-mail: journalscustomerservice-usa@elsevier.com (for print support); journalsonlinesupport-usa@elsevier.com (for online support).**

Reprints. For copies of 100 or more, of articles in this publication, please contact the Commercial Reprints Department, Elsevier Inc., 360 Park Avenue South, New York, NY 10010-1710. Tel. 212-633-3874; Fax: 212-633-3820; E-mail: reprints@elsevier.com.

Physician Assistant Clinics is covered in *EMBASE/Excerpta Medica and ESCI.*

PROGRAM OBJECTIVE
The goal of the Physician Assistant Clinics is to keep practicing physician assistants up to date with current clinical practice by providing timely articles reviewing the state of the art in patient care.

TARGET AUDIENCE
Physician Assistants and other healthcare professionals

LEARNING OBJECTIVES
Upon completion of this activity, participants will be able to:
1. Review the pathophysiology, assessment, evaluation, and management of youth sports-related concussion (SRC).
2. Discuss appropriate diagnosis and management of pediatric idiopathic scoliosis, upper extremity trauma, developmental hip dysplasia, variation in gait, as well as pediatric back and knee pain.
3. Recognize strategies to identify human trafficking victims in a clinical setting while maintaining personal and patient safety.

ACCREDITATION
The Elsevier Office of Continuing Medical Education (EOCME) is accredited by the Accreditation Council for Continuing Medical Education (ACCME) to provide continuing medical education for physicians.

The EOCME designates this journal-based CME activity for a maximum of 10 *AMA PRA Category 1 Credit*(s)™. Physicians should claim only the credit commensurate with the extent of their participation in the activity.

All other healthcare professionals requesting continuing education credit for this enduring material will be issued a certificate of participation.

DISCLOSURE OF CONFLICTS OF INTEREST
The EOCME assesses conflict of interest with its instructors, faculty, planners, and other individuals who are in a position to control the content of CME activities. All relevant conflicts of interest that are identified are thoroughly vetted by EOCME for fair balance, scientific objectivity, and patient care recommendations. EOCME is committed to providing its learners with CME activities that promote improvements or quality in healthcare and not a specific proprietary business or a commercial interest.

The planning committee, staff, authors and editors listed below have identified no financial relationships or relationships to products or devices they or their spouse/life partner have with commercial interest related to the content of this CME activity:
Marcella Andrews, PT, MPT; Jennifer M. Bauer, MD, MS; John Forrest Bennett, MN ARNP; Esther Bennitta; Todd Blumberg, MD; Cora Collette Breuner, MD, MPH, FAAP; Regina Chavous-Gibson, MS, RN; Douglas S. Dedo, PA-C, MCHS; Nicholas Henderson; Katerina Heidhausen; Anju Jain, MS, ATC, PA-C; Ana Maria G. Kolenko, PA-C, MPH; Jeanette Kotch, MA, ATC, PA-C; Keith Lemay, PA-C; Jaclyn Omura, MD; Charity Parenzin; Patrick Parenzin, PA-C; Cheryl Parker, PA-C; Leslie Rodriguez, ATC, PA-C; James A. Van Rhee, MS, PA-C.

UNAPPROVED/OFF-LABEL USE DISCLOSURE
The EOCME requires CME faculty to disclose to the participants:
1. When products or procedures being discussed are off-label, unlabelled, experimental, and/or investigational (not US Food and Drug Administration [FDA] approved); and
2. Any limitations on the information presented, such as data that are preliminary or that represent ongoing research, interim analyses, and/or unsupported opinions. Faculty may discuss information about pharmaceutical agents that is outside of FDA-approved labelling. This information is intended solely for CME and is not intended to promote off-label use of these medications. If you have any questions, contact the medical affairs department of the manufacturer for the most recent prescribing information.

TO ENROLL
The CME program is available to all Physician Assistant Clinics subscribers at no additional fee. To subscribe to the Physician Assistant Clinics, call customer service at 1-800-654-2452 or sign up online at www.physicianassistant.theclinics.com/.

METHOD OF PARTICIPATION
In order to claim credit, participants must complete the following:

1. Complete enrolment as indicated above
2. Read the activity
3. Complete the CME Test and Evaluation. Participants must achieve a score of 70% on the test. All CME Tests and Evaluations must be completed online

CME INQUIRIES/SPECIAL NEEDS

For all CME inquiries or special needs, please contact elsevierCME@elsevier.com.

Contributors

CONSULTING EDITOR

JAMES A. VAN RHEE, MS, PA-C
Associate Professor, Program Director, Yale School of Medicine, Yale Physician Assistant Online Program, New Haven, Connecticut

EDITOR

PATRICK PARENZIN, PA-C
Bachelors of Science, Exercise Physiology, University of Montana, Missoula, Montana; Certificate, Physician Assistant Studies, University of Washington, Department of Pediatric Orthopedics, Seattle Children's Hospital, Seattle, Washington

AUTHORS

MARCELLA ANDREWS, PT, MPT
Physical Therapist, Seattle Children's Hospital, Seattle, Washington

JENNIFER M. BAUER, MD, MS
Seattle Children's Hospital, University of Washington Orthopedics and Sports Medicine, Seattle, Washington

JOHN FORREST BENNETT, MN, ARNP
Nurse Practitioner, Physical Medicine and Rehabilitation, Mary Bridge Children's Hospital, Tacoma, Washington; Affiliate Faculty, University of Washington School of Nursing, Seattle, Washington

TODD BLUMBERG, MD
Medical Doctor, Orthopedics, Seattle Children's Hospital, Seattle, Washington

CORA COLLETTE BREUNER, MD, MPH, FAAP
Professor, Department of Pediatrics, Adolescent Medicine Division, Adjunct Professor, Orthopedics and Sports Medicine, Seattle Children's Hospital, University of Washington, Seattle, Washington

DOUGLAS S. DEDO, PA-C, MCHS
Supervisor of Advanced Practice Providers, Orthopedics and Sports Medicine, Seattle Children's Hospital, Seattle, Washington

ANJU JAIN, MS, ATC, PA-C
Fircrest Rehabilitation Center, Department of Social and Health Services, Shoreline, Washington

ANA MARIA G. KOLENKO, PA-C, MPH
Physician Assistant and First Assist, Orthopedics and Sports Medicine, Seattle Children's Hospital, Seattle, Washington

JEANETTE KOTCH, MA, ATC, PA-C
Physician Assistant, Orthopedics and Sports Medicine, Seattle Children's Hospital, Seattle, Washington

KEITH LEMAY, PA-C
Physician Assistant, Orthopedics, Seattle Children's Hospital, Seattle, Washington

JACLYN OMURA, MD
Acting Assistant Professor, Rehabilitation Medicine, Seattle Children's Hospital, University of Washington School of Medicine, Seattle, Washington

CHARITY PARENZIN
Founder of The America Unchained Project, Guest Educator, Documentarian, Lolo, Montana

PATRICK PARENZIN, PA-C
Bachelors of Science, Exercise Physiology, University of Montana, Missoula, Montana; Certificate, Physician Assistant Studies, University of Washington, Department of Pediatric Orthopedics, Seattle Children's Hospital, Seattle, Washington

CHERYL PARKER, PA-C
Physician Assistant, Orthopedics, Seattle Children's Hospital, Seattle, Washington

LESLIE RODRIGUEZ, PA-C
Physician Assistant, Orthopedics and Sports Medicine, Seattle Children's Hospital, Seattle, Washington

Contents

Foreword: Pediatric Orthopedics xi

James A. Van Rhee

Preface xiii

Patrick Parenzin

How to Identify Human Trafficking Victims in a Clinical Setting 415

Charity Parenzin

Human trafficking is a growing epidemic in the United States. Sex trafficking and the demand for minors—both boys and girls—is on the increase. In this article, Charity Parenzin(i), the founder of The America Unchained Project, uses her years of working with human trafficking survivors, law enforcement officers, and organizational leaders to highlight markers every medical providers should be aware of in order to identify human trafficking victims in a clinical setting and maintain the safety of your patient, yourself, and those around you.

Youth Sports–Related Concussion 431

Anju Jain and Jeanette Kotch

Youth sports–related concussion is first noted with cognitive and somatic symptoms that are transient in nature. The definition of youth sports–related concussion is a functional disturbance to the brain after a blow to the head, neck, or body. Often neuroimaging conducted in the initial evaluation will have negative results. Initial management consists of cognitive and physical rest for a minimum of 48 hours. The return to school protocol should be equally weighted with the return-to-play guidelines for the youth athlete.

Pediatric Idiopathic Scoliosis Diagnosis and Management 441

Ana Maria G. Kolenko and Jennifer M. Bauer

Scoliosis significantly contributes to the burden of pediatric orthopedic deformities. Appropriate diagnosis and management are essential to provide children with the best quality of life in childhood and into adulthood. All providers caring for the pediatric population should be aware of current recommendations as they pertain to pediatric scoliosis.

Pediatric Upper Extremity Trauma 455

Douglas S. Dedo

Arm injuries are an unfortunate by-product of the active lifestyle of a child. This article reviews some of the more common injuries associated with traumatic events and discusses appropriate treatment options. Some injuries are often overtreated, which can cause additional problems such as increased joint stiffness, chronic joint pain, deformity, and extended physical therapy that could potentially be avoided. Some injuries require special attention and longer protection for proper healing and to prevent repeat injuries. This discussion helps to identify these trouble spots to improve the quality of care.

Toe Walking: Review of the Differential Diagnosis and Treatment Options to Ensure Optimal Gross Motor Development   477

John Forrest Bennett and Jaclyn Omura

Toe walking is a common variation in gait in the developing child. The differential for toe walking is broad; therefore, a clinician must approach this gait abnormality with caution. A thorough and intentional history and physical examination can efficiently narrow a differential diagnosis, rule out diagnoses, and guide both diagnostics as well as treatment plans. Treatment of idiopathic toe walking remains controversial.

Hip Dysplasia – Birth to 6 Months   487

Keith Lemay, Cheryl Parker, and Todd Blumberg

 Video content accompanies this article at http://www. physicianassistant.theclinics.com.

Developmental hip dysplasia is the most common musculoskeletal condition affecting newborns. It most commonly affects infants in breech position or those with a family history of hip dysplasia. Early detection starts with an evaluation of hip stability and ultrasound imaging for anyone with an abnormal examination or significant risk factors. Pavlik harness treatment has a high rate of success when initiated early and results in substantial quality of life improvement for patients. Failure to recognize and treat hip dysplasia in an infant results in malformation of the hip joint and leads to early onset hip arthritis.

Anterior Knee Pain in Adolescents: Expanding Your Differential   497

Leslie Rodriguez

Anterior knee pain is among the most common pediatric musculoskeletal complaints. Commonly clinicians attribute this complaint to overuse, inequalities of flexibility and strength, and unique stresses placed on the patellofemoral joint during skeletal growth. Frequent diagnoses include patellofemoral pain syndrome, quadriceps or patella tendinopathy, tibial tubercle apophysitis, pes anserine bursitis, and fat pad impingement. It is important to consider there are less common causes of pediatric anterior knee pain. These may require further workup and specialist referral. Understanding of history taking and physical examination findings is key to forming an accurate working differential diagnoses list and directing timely management.

Adolescent Back Pain   511

Cora Collette Breuner

Back pain is a common complaint in the adolescent population and can affect both the physical and psychological well-being of youth and their families. A thorough history and physical examination can improve early detection and accurate diagnosis. Although underlying serious disorder is rare in adolescents with back pain, health care providers should be familiar with specific signs and symptoms that require decisive evaluation and intervention. This article highlights the significance of combining a thorough history and physical examination in adolescents who present with back pain to steer the initial diagnostic work-up and to improve the accuracy of diagnosis.

Cerebral Palsy: Etiology, Evaluation, and Management of the Most Common Cause for Pediatric Disability   525

John Forrest Bennett, Marcella Andrews, and Jaclyn Omura

Cerebral palsy (CP) is the most common cause of physical disability in childhood. CP is caused by an injury to the developing brain and results in abnormal development of movement and posture. CP has many associated comorbidities, most commonly affecting the musculoskeletal system. Children with CP benefit from early diagnosis, and it is therefore important for the general practitioner to recognize risk factors as well as examination findings suspicious for CP. The impact of CP on the musculoskeletal and nervous systems requires routine surveillance in order to ensure timely interventions occur, in an effort to maximize function.

Toeing, Bowing, and Flatfeet in Children: Kids Come in All Shapes and Sizes   539

Patrick Parenzin

 Video content accompanies this article at http://www. physicianassistant.theclinics.com.

Children's lower extremity shape is exceedingly variable and has a wide range of normal. Flat feet, in-toeing, bowed legs, and knock knees can be normal physiologic variants in the pediatric population. Using a thorough history and basic physical examination, a clinician can determine pathologic deformity versus physiologic variation in the lower extremity of a child.

Pediatric Orthopedics

PHYSICIAN ASSISTANT CLINICS

FORTHCOMING ISSUES

January 2021
Rheumatology
Benjamin Smith, *Editor*

April 2021
Surgery
Courtney Fankhanel, *Editor*

July 2021
Behavioral Health
Kim Zuber and Jane S. Davis, *Editors*

RECENT ISSUES

July 2020
Hospice and Palliative Medicine
Donna Seton and Rich Lamkin, *Editors*

April 2020
Diabetes
Kim Zuber and Jane S. Davis, *Editors*

January 2020
Intrinsic Skills for Physician Assistants
Sharona Kanofsky, *Editor*

SERIES OF RELATED INTEREST

Primary Care: Clinics in Office Practice
https://www.primarycare.theclinics.com/

THE CLINICS ARE AVAILABLE ONLINE!
Access your subscription at:
www.theclinics.com

Foreword

Pediatric Orthopedics

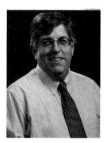

James A. Van Rhee, MS, PA-C
Consulting Editor

According the National Commission on Certification of Physician Assistants *2019 Statistical Profile of Certified Physician Assistants*, 18.7% of all physician assistants work in a surgical subspecialty, and 58% of the physician assistants in surgical subspecialties are in orthopedics.[1] So, while this issue may be of importance to that group, it may play an even more important role to those in primary care and pediatrics, as this issue focuses on pediatric orthopedics.

Guest author Patrick Parenzin has put together a group of knowledgeable authors and topics that are common in the pediatric population and require special attention. Jain and Kotch start the issue off with a review of the evaluation and treatment of adolescent concussion. Bennett covers the musculoskeletal aspects of cerebral palsy. Dedo covers trauma of the upper extremity; Rodriguez presents a review of anterior knee pain, and Parker and Lemay review developmental dysplasia of the hip. Spine and back issues are covered by Kolenko, who covers idiopathic scoliosis, and Bruener, who discusses back pain in the adolescent. This issue also covers foot issues, with Bennett discussing toe walking, and our guest editor reviewing toeing, bowing, and flatfeet in children.

Human trafficking involves the use of force, fraud, or coercion to obtain some type of labor or commercial sex act. Every year, millions of men, women, and children are trafficked worldwide, including the United States. A few years ago, I went to a lecture on human trafficking and met the speaker. Charity Parenzin, the speaker, is the author of the article in this issue on "Human Trafficking: Knowing the Signs." You will find it as eye opening as I did.

Physician Assist Clin 5 (2020) xi–xii
https://doi.org/10.1016/j.cpha.2020.06.011
2405-7991/20/© 2020 Published by Elsevier Inc.

I hope you enjoy this issue. Our next issue will cover rheumatology.

James A. Van Rhee, MS, PA-C
Yale School of Medicine
Yale Physician Assistant Online Program
100 Church Street South, Suite A230
New Haven, CT 06519, USA

E-mail address:
james.vanrhee@yale.edu

Website:
http://www.paonline.yale.edu

REFERENCE

1. National Commission on Certification of Physician Assistants, Inc. April 2020. 2019 Statistical Profile of Certified Physician Assistants: an annual report of the National Commission on Certification of Physician Assistants. Available at: http://www. nccpa.net/research. Accessed June 15, 2020.

Preface

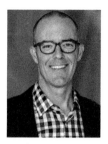

Patrick Parenzin, PA-C
Editor

I have worked with children in one way or another my entire adult life. The titles have been variable: Camp counselor, Coach, Dad, Physician Assistant. But the work is all really quite similar: take care of each kid, teach them pertinent things that you know, and make sure nothing bad happens to them while they are in your care. Easy, right?

Some days the work *is* easy. You are able to work alongside a family in a terrible situation and help fix it. Straighten a bone, explain a difficult medical diagnosis in a way that brings clarity and understanding, recognize a rare condition, expedite treatment. At the end of the day you have done the work: you've taken care of a child, you've taught them what you know, and, most importantly, you've protected them from further harm.

Then there are other days. The hard days. In reality, these days are few and far between, but (for various psychological reasons that my orthopedic brain cannot comprehend) you think of them often. Often they weigh on you. Perhaps you have had similar days. Those days where every child you are treating screams as you walk in the room. Every family seems confused and upset with your explanations. The day you missed a significant diagnosis....something bad happened and you weren't able to stop it.

And yet, despite the frustrations and demands, off to the next room you go. Room after room. Then, a break in the hard. Behind one door you find a 4-year-old boy dressed like Spider-man. His cast (from the open both-bone forearm fracture) is painted to look like a web thrower. He practices his web-spinning skills on you. And your hard day just got a lot less laborious. Joy has filled the room as Spider-man has come to lighten the load as all good heroes do.

Kids are incredible. They demonstrate what it means to adapt. They often find joy where no one else could. (A cast on a broken bone? No way! That's a web thrower!) They are unscripted, wonderfully loud, joyful balls of incredible tenacity. And their gifts and value often go overlooked by most of society.

Children are the most precious resources on planet earth, and those who have come together to write the articles in the following pages are doing everything they can to protect this resource daily. Together they bring a diverse cornucopia of experience

Physician Assist Clin 5 (2020) xiii–xiv
https://doi.org/10.1016/j.cpha.2020.06.010
2405-7991/20/© 2020 Published by Elsevier Inc.

physicianassistant.theclinics.com

and clinical expertise, which they have contributed to this issue. My hope is that you are able to learn from each contributor's writing. However, what I hope will inspire you is not so much what they have written, but the excellence of care they bring to each child and family they care for as a provider or educator. They take care of the kid AND the family. They teach them what they know AND they teach legions of other providers. They make sure nothing bad happens to children, and they also try to make sure you can do the same.

As Physician Assistants, it is our goal to care for others. It is also our goal to inspire lifelong health and learning. However, to see it in action is a whole other thing. So, it is with that in mind that I say a huge thank you to each of the authors and to you the reader. We as providers get to do the best work in the world—some days easy, some days hard. Each day caring for our most precious natural resource: our children.

Patrick Parenzin, PA-C
Department of Pediatric Orthopedics
Seattle Children's Hospital
4800 Sandpoint Way NE
OA.9.120.1 PO Box 5371
Seattle, WA 98145-5005, USA

E-mail address:
patrick.parenzin@seattlechildrens.org

How to Identify Human Trafficking Victims in a Clinical Setting

Charity Parenzin

KEYWORDS

- Human trafficking education • Identify • Sexual abuse • CME

KEY POINTS

- According to a study published in the Annuals of Health Law, 87.7% of all human trafficking victims in the United States will see a medical provider during captivity. This means that providers and staff have opportune time to help facilitate a potential rescue for victims.
- It is of utmost importance for providers to realize that they are each one of many people whose actions of compassion and care, when added together, can lead to a safe and hopeful rescue.
- Understanding the difference between prostitution and human trafficking is clear if you understand the signs.
- There are key physical, emotional, and mental signs of human trafficking that can lead providers and staff to identify potential human trafficking victims while they are in clinic.
- Children can be exploited by others while still in the home. Making parents aware of the vulnerability of tween and teens is important for keeping children safe.

IDENTIFYING HUMAN TRAFFICKING VICTIMS IN A CLINICAL SETTING

According to Homeland Security in the United States, "Human trafficking involves the use of force, fraud, or coercion to obtain some type of labor or commercial sex act. Every year, millions of men, women, and children are trafficked worldwide, including right here in the United States. It can happen in any community and victims can be of any age, race, gender, or nationality. Traffickers might use violence, manipulation, or false promises of well-paying jobs or romantic relationships to lure victims into trafficking situations."[1]

Human trafficking in the United States is growing in both demand and awareness. As these factors increase, people from all walks of life are often left wondering what they can do to play a part in the rescue of people forced to live a life of constant

c/o The Lifeguard Group, 111 N Higgins Ave #417, Missoula, MT 59802, USA
E-mail address: charity@americaunchained.org
Twitter: @parenzini (C.P.)

Physician Assist Clin 5 (2020) 415–430
https://doi.org/10.1016/j.cpha.2020.06.008
2405-7991/20/© 2020 Elsevier Inc. All rights reserved.

fear and mental and physical trauma. Although everyone can prioritize self-education about signs of human trafficking, there are key groups of professionals who can make a significant difference in this fight for freedom. Those key groups include law enforcement, medical professionals, and teachers.

As mandated reporters and trained crisis professionals, these groups are poised to identify, report, and rescue individuals as part of their professional mandate. In addition, these groups are highly engaged in the population who is the most vulnerable to victimization—minors. This creates a unique point of view and opportunity most other professions do not have. It is this vantage point that empowers these professionals the potential to be a part of the rescue of hundreds or even thousands of individuals across the United States who are being trafficked everyday.

In addition to their unique vantage point and capability to rescue those in danger, medical providers, specifically, hold a key advantage above other professionals: access. According to a study published in the Annuals of Health Law, 87.7% of all human trafficking victims in the United States will see a medical provider during captivity.[2] And, of those patients, 97% explain they were not offered assistance out of their situation or identified as a victim of human trafficking.[3] This means that most of all human trafficking victims are coming into hospitals and clinics for treatment while still in the confines of their captor only to leave and go back to the same life as before. However, if providers and staff are made aware of signs that indicate trafficking, they can allow time to help facilitate a potential rescue for victims.

THE FACE OF HUMAN TRAFFICKING IN THE UNITED STATES

For the purposes of this article, we cannot delve into the full scale of human trafficking in the United States; however, it is important to understand a general overview of the problem. With this understanding, one can better understand that each person in the fight has a valuable role to play. And, in a sinister battle where there are many players, every person empowered to rescue victims is vital to changing the course of this war.

Estimates for human trafficking victims vary greatly given that victims are often unfound or unreported with only about 0.04% survivors of human trafficking cases identified as such.[4] Internationally it is estimated that there are between 20 million and 40 million people trafficked everyday. Grasping the full scope of this human trafficking is highly challenging because so many cases are undetected, making it an issue referred to by the United Nations as "the hidden figure of crime."[5,6]

In the United States, the current estimate of people being trafficked varies between absolutes and estimates, due to the aforementioned lack of reporting, identification, and understanding. These numbers range widely—from 250,000 to more than 400,000—[7] and include both sex and labor trafficking, men and women, adults and children, foreign nationals, and US citizens. Specifically in reported sex trafficking cases to the FBI, it was found that

- 94% of reported victims are women
- 83% are US citizens
- 64% of cases involved the commercial exploitation of a minor

The FBI and Special Task Forces have also discovered that the average age for children to enter the commercial sex trade is 12 to 14 years for girls and 11 to 13 years for boys, making the issue of sex trafficking one that reaches some of the most vulnerable in our population.[8–10] However bothersome, these data are important to keep in mind when assessing the potential abuse of any patient. It is also key to note that many of these children are frequently trafficked by someone who seems to have a personal relationship with them (or by someone who seems to be in their lives regularly). People who are or who claim to be relatives, a parent's significant other, and family friends may be involved in sexual transactions involving a child who is being trafficked—especially if they are being trafficking out of their own home. This revelation might help dislodge the notion that only circuit criminals are involved in trafficking children, allowing for providers to better identify victims.

THE DOMINO EFFECT

When dealing with a potential victim of human trafficking, you need to remember that many of them will see various medical providers during their captivity (**Fig. 1**). This means that you most likely have not been the first nor will you be the last person from which they will seek medical attention. With this in mind, it is of utmost importance for you to realize that you are one of many people whose actions of compassion and care, when added together, can lead to a safe and hopeful rescue. Essentially, your interactions are one part of building a bridge to freedom for a person trapped in a living nightmare.

For some medical providers, this realization can be hopeful, knowing that you can play a part in leading someone out of mental, emotional, and physical bondage. For others it can be more of a disappointment, as some are led to believe that they alone can be the sole rescuer of any human trafficking victim. (One that gallantly seems to free someone from their life of misery). In either case, it is important to face the reality of the situation—you are not alone.

The truth is, although every rescue of a human trafficking victim is done so by a person (or group of persons) who took action, it is likely that that moment is the culmination of several, if not dozens, of previous interactions with other professionals, including other medical providers. Every person's part is vital in securing the safety and rescue of human trafficking victims. This is by all accounts a team effort. And, if everyone does their part, more victims will be led out of the captivity they are currently living. When we begin to see our interactions as part of a whole, it is less overwhelming and often less discouraging.

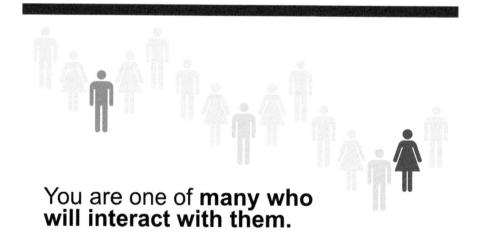

You are one of **many who will interact with them.**

Fig. 1. Many health care providers will interact with human trafficking victims during the course of their captivity. You are one of many. (*Courtesy of* The America Unchained Project.)

Most human trafficking victims are controlled by fear, lies, substances, or all of the above-mentioned. Their mindset is not in a place of clear logic or rationale. This means they will likely not trust you or anyone else to keep them safe if they are meeting you for the first time. It will probably take time and frequent healthy interactions to build trust of any person, institution, or profession.

Often, when initially offered safety and resources, victims of human trafficking reject the offer and stay in captivity. However, if you have played your part in giving them the medical attention they need while treating them with dignity and respect, you can be confident that your interaction with them has left a positive impression. An impression that, when added together with others like it, can lead to a rescue in the future. Again, know your part is vital, even if you do not see the "happily ever after" ending you hope will come in the moment.

SEX WORK VERSUS SEX TRAFFICKING

Many clinicians are concerned about the differences between prostitution and human trafficking, stating that the lines are often blurred. They want to be respectful and non-judgmental, but they also wish to protect those in their care. For this reason it is important to acquaint yourself with the clear delineations between a sex work and human trafficking.

First, it is important to note that sex work is illegal in all states and all but one county in the country. And, although no provider would ever want to vilify a patient, knowing that illegal activity is present does open your patient to risks that can put them in dangerous situations regardless of victimization. With that in mind, the differences between chosen sex work as an income source and someone who is being trafficked is as follows:

- Sex workers have voluntary involvement; human trafficking victims do not
- Sex workers work independently or with a pimp; human trafficking victims always have a pimp or trafficker
- Sex workers stay in the same geographic location; victims of human trafficking move locations
- Sex workers are paid; human trafficking victims are not
- Sex work may be illegal or legal; trafficking is always illegal
- Sex workers are not controlled through fraud, force, or coercion; trafficking involves force, fraud, or coercion

In all of this, it is of primary importance to remember that ALL minors involved in commercial sex acts are victims of human trafficking regardless of state or county statues concerning sex work. If you suspect any minor of being commercially trafficked or trafficked out of their home, report this immediately to the authorities. They are not workers; they are victims in need of rescue.

LOOKING PAST WHAT YOU EXPECT

In the past 15 years, a plethora of media has been created to portray the world of human trafficking and its victims. From television shows to movies, documentaries to high-adrenaline action films, these representations of human trafficking (especially sex trafficking) are dramatic and intense. However, although elements of those movies ring true, they are by no means the full picture of the pool of actual victims. The idea of being from another country, crossing international territories, traveling constantly, or having freedom to choose another occupation is one of many misconceptions portrayed in fictional representations of human trafficking. For this reason, it is important you look past what you *think* you should expect when assessing someone. When seen through the correct lens, their abuses could lead to the identification of human trafficking.

One common misconception is that victims of sex trafficking are often from other countries, smuggled into the United States on crates or boats as cargo. Or they are flown here on false work visas. Although situations of foreign persons being brought here for trafficking do occur, most victims of sex trafficking in the United States are citizens born in the United States. In fact, most are never trafficked internationally—before or after they are brought into the life.

Furthermore, many victims who are in the United States come out of the foster care system. According to the US Department of State, "Recent reports have consistently indicated that a large number of victims of child sex trafficking were at one time in the foster care system."[3] This is valuable to note, as many providers will work with such vulnerable populations.

Again, anyone being threatened, coerced, held captive through addiction or otherwise, or fraudulently kept in debt in exchange for sex acts are indeed victims of human trafficking. As a provider, you must treat them as such. Once identified these women, men, and children can be given the opportunity to embrace freedom and rehabilitation. By knowing the difference between myth and reality, providers are one step closer to rescuing more people out of human trafficking.

TYPES OF CLINICS WHERE VICTIMS SEEK MEDICAL CARE

Human trafficking victims can see medical providers in a variety of clinical settings, and often more than one clinical setting is visited by a victim during their captivity. The chart in **Fig. 2** shows the breakdown of types of clinics victims said they visited while being trafficked.[1] With this information in mind, providers and their staff can better equip their clinic on protocols and safety should a suspected victim be seen in their facility.

LAYERED HEALTH SYMPTOMS

The 4 most common reasons that present in a victim of human sex trafficking are sleep deprivation or sleep disorders, workplace injuries, sexually transmitted infection (STI), and urinary tract infection. However, these are not the only indicators by far. In one study, 57% of trafficked victims had 12 or more concurrent health symptoms at the

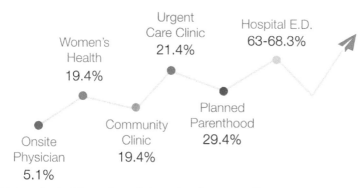

Fig. 2. This is a chart of the various clinic settings human trafficking survivors said they went to during their captivity. (*Courtesy of* The America Unchained Project.)

time of discovery[11,12] (**Fig. 3**). This fact is important to note because, as you learn more indicators, you will be able to connect layered health symptoms as a potential identification tool.

PHYSICAL AND VERBAL INDICATORS OF HUMAN TRAFFICKING

This is the part of the article where you will be requested to participate in an interactive activity. If time and location allows, please find access to the Internet. It might be your phone, on your computer, or on your tablet.

Once online, please search the phrase "Human Trafficking Tattoo" into your search engine. (I apologize if this affects your otherwise pristine search history). Now, pay attention to what you are seeing. Note names, symbols, and phrases. Also note the locations on the body the tattoo is placed. These nuances are important to be made aware of as you might very well see them again in a clinical setting. (Or, as I have learned when doing live presentations, you might have already seen such tattoos but did not know what it was you were witnessing).

With this new knowledge, what otherwise would have been something you passed by, is now something that makes you take note. That said, there are many physical indicators of human trafficking. In movies, these are usually denoted by obvious markings of trauma and physical abuse. But, in reality, they are not always that easy to spot. The first clear indicator, if present, is often that of the aforementioned tattoo (**Fig. 4**). These can appear on various parts of the body, including the mouth, chest, neck, lower back, and vulva. However, many other physical and verbal indicators (some of which are explored in more detail later in this article) may also be present such as the following[13–18]:

- Physical signs of trauma
- Unexplained or conflicting story
- Inappropriate dress for weather conditions
- Usage of terminology from the life
- Lack of control of own finances

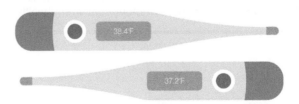

"In one study, fifty-seven percent (57%) of trafficked victims had 12 or more concurrent health symptoms at the time of discovery." (6)

Fig. 3. Human trafficking victims frequently present with a large number of various health symptoms. (*Courtesy of* The America Unchained Project.)

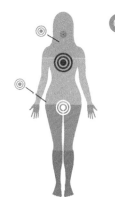

01   Tattoo in specific locations:

- Mouth
- Chest
- Neck
- Lower back
- Vulva

Fig. 4. Tattoos are a common form of ID on human trafficking victims. This image lists the common locations you will find such tattoos. (*Courtesy of* The America Unchained Project.)

When evaluating a patient, if you witness these indicators, take note. You may also need to mentally switch gears because what you may have initially thought you were going to treat could quickly escalate into something far more complicated. Naturally, you will want to treat the issue for which the patient has come to you. However, be prepared to treat a myriad of other problems as well, including that of a someone who most likely is in dire need of safety.

LANGUAGE AND TERMS FROM "THE LIFE"

Another indication that can red flag a suspicion that someone is a victim of human trafficking is language. Pay attention to the type of words they use when talking about their line of work or daily routines. Often, persons being trafficked will use terms from what is known as "the life." And, even if they are being forced or coerced to do their "job," they will see it as just that, a job. In fact, most women trafficked in the sex trade are convinced that they are there by a series of their own choices, or that they made a series of bad decisions that ultimately got them to where they are. Because of this, despite violence, abuse, neglect, and often starvation, women frequently discuss job-related activities in a very matter-of-fact nature. In turn, they usually respond to matter-of-fact lines of questioning with ease. For this reason, it is important to be aware of terms frequently used, as their use can be key indicators that they are, indeed, victims of sex trafficking.

The following are a few terms and phrases from "the life" most often used to describe events or processes in their line of work. For a full list of terminology you can visit The America Unchained Project's Website (https://www.americaunchained.net/resources) and sign up to receive our free resources, which includes a more extensive list of terms from the life.

Key words to be made aware of are as follows:

- Circuit Girl—a prostitute who moves around the country working
- Daddy—a term prostitutes use for their pimps
- Date—act of prostitution with John or Trick

- Game/Bizz—a term pimp uses for his work
- Lace/Lace Up—when a pimp gives his prostitute clothing or schooling
- L.E. —Law Enforcement
- Mac—a pimp who participates in other criminal activity; a master of corruption
- Out of Pocket—when a prostitute changes pimps
- Party—act of prostitution
- Trick/John—a man who pays for sex

Particular things to note in their use of language are slang, phrases, labels for people in their life, and colorful words for sex acts (**Fig. 5**). You can often illicit the use of personal terminology by asking key questions about their daily habits, friends and family, or work environment. Knowing language commonly used in "the life" is one step closer to helping identify and rescue victims of human trafficking.

ADDITIONAL BEHAVIORS TO CONSIDER

In our every changing world of communication, it can be hard to note patterns of talk or behavior that are bothersome when there is often such a short amount of time with each patient. However, being aware of unusual behaviors during an interaction will help guide you to recognize potential concerns. Some behaviors include lack of eye contact, being in a hurry to leave, checking their phone frequently, forgetting details when asked the same questions more than once, and not knowing their location, day of the week, or date. In addition to physical and verbal indicators, these actions are clues that the patient is most likely living a very risky life, one that might be human trafficking.[13–18]

EMOTIONAL INDICATORS

When evaluating patients for sexual abuse there are emotion and/or mental indicators that help alert medical personnel that there is need for intervention. However, when

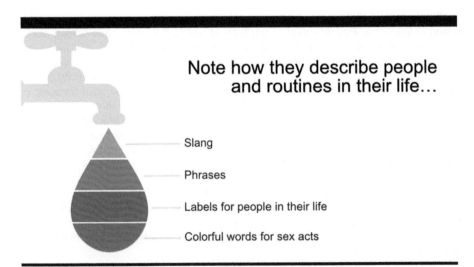

Fig. 5. Conversation and terminology are a good indicator that someone maybe involved in human trafficking. This image shows 4 key conversational methods to take note of when talking with someone you suspect may be a victim of human trafficking. (*Courtesy of* The America Unchained Project.)

abuses delve into the realm of human sex trafficking, those indicators often increase in intensity and frequency. Although we cannot discuss each one in depth, be aware of those that present the most often.

When dealing with a potential victim of human sex trafficking, the patient might present symptoms of the following:

- Anxiety/hypervigilance/panic attacks
- Depressed mood/flat affect
- Somatization
- Posttraumatic stress disorder
- Memory disruption
- Emotional dysregulation
- Trauma bonding

Again, keep in mind, the above-mentioned symptoms are not the only emotional indicators for human trafficking. But they are the ones that present most frequently. Human trafficking victims are not good emotional regulators, as their life does not promote health on any level. This dysregulation can cause irrational behavior. Learning to identify it as symptomatic of a potentially deeper issue is a step forward in identification and rescue.[13–18]

REPRODUCTIVE HEALTH INDICATORS OF POTENTIAL VICTIMS

One key to identifying sex trafficking victims is to recognize that their reproductive health indicators will be highly irregular. It is important to also note that there may be one or more of these indicators present and these symptoms may not be the reason they have come to your clinic for treatment. Finally, most victims will give varying excuses for treatment that can mask deeper, more complex issues. For these reasons, you must always be willing to take time with anyone you suspect has experienced sexual abuse or trafficking, as their symptoms may help lead you to reveal a deeper issue in their lives.

With this in mind, the common reproductive health indicators facing potential victims (as indicated in **Fig. 6**) include the following:

- Multiple or recurrent STIs
- Abnormally high number of sexual partners
- Trauma to the vagina or rectum
- Pregnancy at a young age

SIGNS OF SEXUAL EXPLOITATION IN MINORS

When dealing with minors, it is important to note that any and all sexual exploitation is considered human trafficking. There are no gray lines here. In addition, it is key to note that minors are often swayed by highly dramatic, often emotionally-intoxicating scenarios. They will frequently paint their lives to be very different from reality. And, to blur lines of indication even more, they are sometimes being trafficked while still at home—by a relative, friend, boyfriend, or girlfriend.

Keeping this in mind, the following are some key indications of sexual exploitation in minors[18] (**Figs. 7–9**).

- Evidence of controlling or dominating relationships
- Signs of physical or sexual abuse
- Signs of drugs or alcohol use
- Pregnancy at a young age

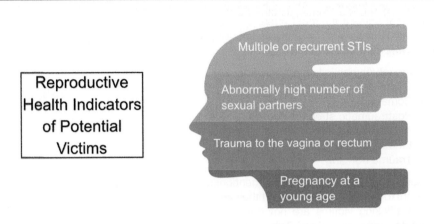

Fig. 6. Reproductive health indicators are a central anchor to identifying someone as a potential victim of human trafficking. The above image lists some of those that are key to note. (*Courtesy of* The America Unchained Project.)

- Evidence of abortions at a young age
- Early sex initiation
- Abnormal number of sexual partners for a young age
- History of running away from home or foster care placements
- Truancy/stops attending school
- Highly sexualized behavior or dress
- Angry or aggressive with staff

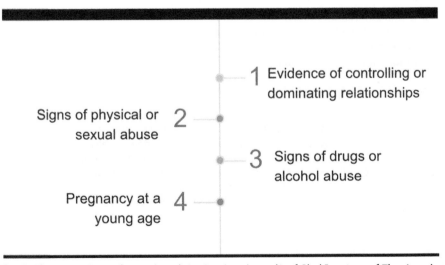

Fig. 7. These are signs of sexual exploitation in minors (1 of 3). (*Courtesy of* The America Unchained Project.)

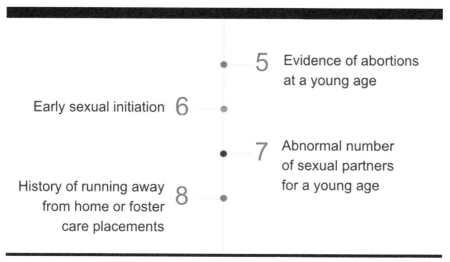

Fig. 8. These are signs of sexual exploitation in minors (2 of 3).

IMPORTANT SCREENING QUESTIONS TO REMEMBER

Because so many minors experience trafficking and exploitation while still living at home, or they are groomed while still living at home, it is important to seek out the level of vulnerability of minors in your care. Parental involvement in this is key, albeit sometimes hard to broach as a topic. However, including screening questions during a visit will help you better assess potential vulnerabilities, allowing you to follow-up as needed.

When talking with a minor or their parent, there are important screening questions to remember. With these questions, you can better gauge if a child is being exploited or is

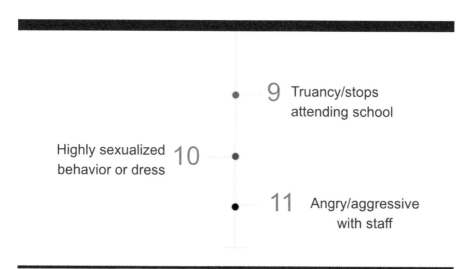

Fig. 9. These are signs of sexual exploitation in minors (3 of 3). (*Courtesy of* The America Unchained Project.)

vulnerable to victimization. For this reason, *The America Unchained Project* offers a downloadable PDF of such questions on our Website. In addition, several are listed later to help assist you in evaluating a patient.

Keep in mind, when you interact with a minor or their parent (or both) the goal is to get the conversation flowing naturally. Do not layer questions about behavior, relationships, or other red-flag indicators together. This may alarm your patient or their guardian. It may also illicit an insincere response. Instead, alternate screening questions with conventional topics to create a simple free-flow nature of how you introduce them. Finally, begin with open-ended questions. If there is cause for concern, you can then adjust your line of questions to closed-ended (yes or no) questions.[19]

That said, here are some questions that are important to ask in order to get a good assessment of if a minor might be vulnerable to or participating in human trafficking:

What/Who Are Their Adult Relationships?

Children should not have adult relationships that are not monitored by their parent or guardian. Distant adult relatives or any adult who has a personal relationship with the child should only do so with the express permission and transparency of the parent. Secret adult relationships are a red-flag.

What Is the Capacity of Their Online Presence?

Online presence for minors should be highly limited and monitored by the parent. Despite a child's desire for adult-level privacy, it is absolutely inappropriate and can create extreme vulnerability for the child or teenager. Parents should be made aware of the fact that people prey on children online frequently—both strangers and those who may know the child or family personally. Parents need to limit their children's online presence with the use of filters and keeping up with their interactions.

Who Are Their Friends of Friends (Kids the Parent Do Not Know)? How Often Are They Around Them?

Parents should know who their kids are around regularly. Friends of friends can be an easy way to introduce children and teens to online vulnerability or people who may wish to harm them. It is imperative that children and teens' parents know who their kids are hanging around.

Who Do They Interact with on a Regular Basis? Does the Parent Know Them?

In addition to friends of friends, often kids and teens hang out with large groups of people away from home. School trips, sports teams, youth group… any large group of kids has people whom mom and dad may not know. It is important to assess if there are groups of people—children or adults—with which the patient is in regular contact.

Are They Afforded Adult-Level Privacy?

It cannot be overstated that privacy is a key element of vulnerability to exploitation. Children and teens who are given adult-level privacy are much more likely to be victimized. The standard rule of thumb given by many law enforcement and FBI task force members who assist in public awareness education, and the location and rescue of human trafficking victims, is that no child or teen should be allowed Internet access in their room on any device at any time. This means that kids and teens text, email, and surf online in the public domain of their house only. Even if the child or teen gives push back, or the parent is resistant to this request, reiterate that adult-level privacy is not appropriate for nonadults. Despite their maturity level, children allowed adult-level

Internet access are far more vulnerable to being preyed on, bullied, and otherwise victimized.

HOW TO POSTURE YOURSELF WHEN INTERACTING WITH A POTENTIAL VICTIM OF SEX TRAFFICKING

When interacting with a patient you suspect is a victim of sex trafficking, it is important you are aware of power dynamics and your overall presence. Human trafficking victims are highly perceptive of body language and tone. They survive by knowing how to read people. And they are reading you from their first interaction. Therefore you should be aware of how you present yourself to them. The way in which you present your mannerisms, use of terminology, tonality, and general attitude can add up to a successful interaction. And each successful interaction with a trusted medical professional is one step closer to this person being led out of trafficking and into safety.

When posturing yourself, note your physical stance. The focus should be to be on their level, not in a domineering position looking down on them. Try to make eye contact, but, remember, most human trafficking victims of any age are not comfortable making eye contact. I have personally worked with several who have shared with me that making direct eye contact is very difficult even now, years after they were rescued. For many reasons, eye contact creates a feeling of fear or shame and they will most likely avoid direct eye contact for a long period of time or all together. However, regardless of them returning eye contact, you should remain in a position of what would be seen as equality, seated on their level whenever possible.

Another consideration when talking to patients is to talk on their level. Talking in terminology that is laden in medical terms or otherwise can leave anyone feeling demeaned, patronized, or even unintelligent. Although many of these women and men are stunted in their education, they are not incapable of understanding. Simply adjust your vocabulary to be confident and inclusive. This will help build trust as they will be better apt to understand everything you are discussing with them.

Naturally coinciding with vocabulary is your tone of voice. Whether desired or not, tonality can impress on people far more than the words you say. Adjusting your tone can make a difference in how you are perceived as well as what people will hear you communicate. Be aware of any tone that is potentially construed as arrogant, rude, or dismissive and make adjustments accordingly. Instead, strive to be patient and calm. Even if you use few words in your interaction, make sure that those words are delivered with the intent of understanding the situation and connecting with your patient.

Finally, be aware of how you present yourself to patients (I like to call it "keep your attitude in check"). Many work environments are run with a fast pace and crowded schedule. Add potential sleep deprivation to the mix and anyone's bedside manner can suffer. However, when attitude is perceived as demeaning or disrespectful, you will quickly lose any hope of forming a connection or building trust with a patient who is in need of safety. Take time to mentally readjust your attitude whenever possible. This action, alongside how you stand, the words you use, and your tone will insure the best possible interaction with your patient (**Fig. 10**).

CREATING A FEELING OF SAFETY AND CONFIDENCE

When trying to bridge a relationship with someone whom you suspect is being trafficking, there are key actions you can learn to take that will assist in reaching this goal. However, even if you learn and use these actions, it is important to keep in

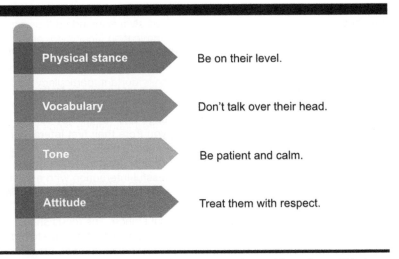

Fig. 10. Be aware of your communication during interactions with patients. This image highlights simple ways in which you can alter your body language and tone to better put your patient at ease. (*Courtesy of* The America Unchained Project.)

mind that human trafficking victims live in a world of someone else's lies (**Fig. 11**). They are not "living" in the reality you and I know to be true.

Traffickers thrive on painting a false reality of fear and doubt in the minds of their victims. What may seem obvious and trustworthy to you may be something victims do not trust in any way. And, in order to break through these lies, you should seek to create a feeling of safety and confidence in your words, actions, and posturing.

Establishing a feeling of safety can be very simple if you follow the following steps:

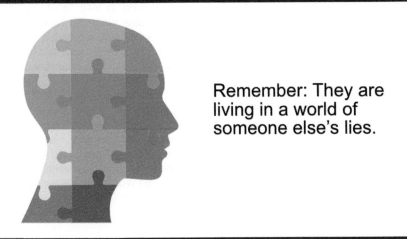

Remember: They are living in a world of someone else's lies.

Fig. 11. It is always good to be reminded that victims of human trafficking (both sex trafficking and labor trafficking) are living in a world of lies. (*Courtesy of* The America Unchained Project.)

- Meet their basic needs (do not overthink it).
- Build rapport. Talk to them with dignity and respect.
- Be conscious of body language and terminology.
- Be sensitive to power dynamics. Give them their power back.
- Always offer water. Simple kindness builds a bridge.
- Reassure them they are safe. Be confident but do not overpromise.

Meeting basic needs is a first step to helping human trafficking victims. They often work all night at the whims and pleasures of others. Simple things such as regular food and water are luxuries not often afforded them. They are surviving, not thriving. So, offering simple necessities helps build trust. Anything more and they suspect you want something from them — a normal expectation in their world.

In addition to meeting basic needs, realize that these victims are not treated with dignity and respect. They are controlled by people who use them, even if they truly think they are being loved. By showing them they have worth through your interactions — your rapport, body language, and power dynamics — you can gain their trust.

Finally, reassure them that they are safe. Do not overpromise heroic acts of rescue, but let them know if they ever wanted out of their situation, your hospital or clinic is a place they can come. Even if they do not seem to believe you or refuse to stay and seek help, you are planting a scenario of hope in their minds that can be useful if and when they choose to leave.

YOU ARE MAKING A DIFFERENCE

Remember that by learning how to better identify human trafficking victims you are allowing yourself to be at the forefront of this fight. We encourage you to tell others about this article and our free online resources so that they can also learn. The more people who are empowered to learn about identifying human trafficking victims the more victims will be rescued. If we all play our part, the idea of freedom for everyone in the United States in our lifetime is possible.

DISCLOSURE

The authors have nothing to disclose.

REFERENCES

1. The U.S. Department of Homeland Security, What is Human Trafficking. 2020. Available at: https://www.dhs.gov/blue-campaign/what-human-trafficking. Accessed February, 2020.
2. Lederer L. The Health Consequences of Sex Trafficking and Their Implications for Identifying Victims in Healthcare Facilities. Ann Health Law 2014;23:61.
3. Coalition to Abolish Slavery and Trafficking. (2017). Identification and referral in health care settings. Available at: http://www.castla.org/assets/files/identification_and_referral_in_health_care_settings_survey_report_vjen.pdf. Accessed April, 2018.
4. What is Human Trafficking." Californians Against Sexual Exploitation. Available at: http://www.caseact.org/learn/humantrafficking/. Accessed July 31, 2019.
5. "Forced Labor, Modern Slavery, and Human Trafficking." International Labor Organization. Available at: http://www.ilo.org/global/topics/forced-labour/lang–en/index.htm. Accessed July 31, 2019.

6. "Monitoring Target 16.2 of the United Nations Sustainable Development Goals." United Nations Office on Drug and Crime. Available at: https://www.unodc.org/documents/research/UNODC-DNR_research_brief.pdf. Accessed July 31, 2018.

7. "Country studies: the United States", the global slavery index. 2020. Available at: https://www.globalslaveryindex.org/2018/findings/country-studies/united-states/. Accessed March, 2018.

8. United States Department of State. 2019 Trafficking in Persons Report - United States of America. 2019. Available at: https://www.state.gov/reports/2019-trafficking-in-persons-report/. Accessed December, 2019.

9. "Human Trafficking Within and Into The United States: A Review of the Literature." Office of the Assistant Secretary for Planning and Evaluation. Available at: https://aspe.hhs.gov/report/human-trafficking-and-within-united-states-review-literature#Trafficking. Accessed July 31, 2019.

10. Schwarz C, Unruh E, Cronin K, et al. Human Trafficking Identification and Service Provision in the Medical and Social Service Sectors. Health Hum Rights 2016;18(1):181–92.

11. IPATH Taskforce, Indiana Protection for Abused and Trafficked Humans. Available at: https://icesaht.org/human-trafficking/ipath-taskforce/. Accessed February, 2018.

12. Baker, Guy Police Detective & Task Force Officer on FBI Safe Streets Task Force, (personal interview), December 2018.

13. Macy RJ, Graham LM. Identifying domestic and international sex-trafficking victims during human service provision. Trauma Violence Abuse 2012;13(2):59–76.

14. Alpert EJ, Ahn R, Albright E, et al. Human trafficking: guidebook on identification, assessment, and response in the health care setting. Boston: MGH Human Trafficking Initiative, Division of Global Health and Human Rights, Department of Emergency Medicine, Massachusetts General Hospital; 2014. Committee on Violence Intervention and Prevention, Massachusetts Medical Society, Waltham, MA.

15. Bessell S, Baldwin SB, Vandenberg ME, et al. Human trafficking and health care providers: lessons learned from federal criminal indictments and civil trafficking cases. Human Trafficking Legal Center and HEAL Trafficking; 2017.

16. Stoklosa H, Beth Dawson M, Williams-Oni F, et al. A Review of U.S. health care institution protocols for the identification and treatment of victims of human trafficking. J Hum Traffick 2017;3(2):116–24.

17. Altun S, Abas M, Zimmerman C, et al. Mental health and human trafficking: responding to survivors' needs. Bjpsych Int 2017;14(1):21–3.

18. Institute of Medicine and National Research Council. Confronting commercial sexual exploitation and sex trafficking of minors in the United States: a guide for providers of victim and support services. Washington, DC: The National Academies Press; 2014. https://doi.org/10.17226/18798.

19. Monroe County Department of Human Services. Screening questions for routine intake assessment. 2019. Available at: www.dorightbykids.org. Accessed December, 2019.

Youth Sports–Related Concussion

Anju Jain, MS, ATC, PA-C[a], Jeanette Kotch, MA, ATC, PA-C[b],*

KEYWORDS

- Youth sports–related concussion • Youth concussion evaluation
- Youth concussion management

KEY POINTS

- Youth sports–related concussion occurs with a functional disturbance rather than a structural injury to the brain after a blow to the head, neck, or body.
- Cognitive and somatic signs or symptoms in patients younger than 18 years may take up to 4 weeks to resolve.
- Initial evaluation via neuroimaging is usually negative.
- Initial management consists of cognitive and physical rest.
- Return-to-school protocol should be prioritized over return-to-play guidelines.

INTRODUCTION

Youth sports–related concussion is an important topic in the return-to-play criteria due to the lack of adolescent-focused long-term studies that demonstrate the prolonged effects of concussion. The incidence of concussion on an annual basis in the United States is approximately 1.7 to 1.8 million, per the data from the Centers for Disease Control.[1] These numbers of incidences for concussion annually are most likely underreported. The actual incidence of concussion is most likely much higher. The incidence of concussion occurring in different sports has a gender delineation. The incidence for concussion in boys is the highest in football, wrestling, and ice hockey.[2] The incidence for concussion in girls is the highest in soccer, lacrosse, and basketball, with the girls' rate of incidents equal to or greater than the rate reported in boys.[2]

DEFINITION OF CONCUSSION

The understanding of a concussion varies from provider to provider. A sports-related concussion is defined as an impact to the head or a whiplash motion in which the brain

[a] Fircrest Rehabilitation Center, Department of Social and Health Services, 15230 15th Avenue NE, Shoreline, WA 98155, USA; [b] Orthopedics and Sports Medicine, Seattle Children's Hospital, 4800 Sand Point Way Northeast OA 9.120, Seattle, WA 98105, USA
* Corresponding author.
E-mail address: jeanette.kotch@seattlechildrens.org

Physician Assist Clin 5 (2020) 431–440
https://doi.org/10.1016/j.cpha.2020.06.003
2405-7991/20/© 2020 Elsevier Inc. All rights reserved.

hits the backside of the skull, creating an injury to the function of the brain.[3] In most concussions, there are no injuries to the structures of the brain. The injury reflects a functional disturbance rather than structural injury to the brain.[3] An analogy that can be used equates the brain to the hardware of a computer. A sports-related concussion is a software injury not a hardware injury. Therefore, initial imaging studies such as a computed tomography (CT) scan often have negative findings for structural deficits.[3]

Sports-related concussion also fits under the category of traumatic brain injury (TBI) due to the symptoms that can be immediate and transient.[3] Furthermore, a concussion is considered a mild TBI noting the umbrella term that denotes injury to the brain, which is vague in terms of specific mechanism of injury and not validated. The following are the definitions of sports-related concussion based on the fifth International Conference on Concussion in Sport Berlin Guidelines from October 2016[3]:

- "Sports related concussion: the immediate and transient symptoms of traumatic brain injury"[3]
- "Sports related concussion is a brain injury, induced by biomechanical forces"[3]
- "Caused by blows that are directly administered to the head, face, neck, or elsewhere on the body"[3]
- "Can have an 'impulsive' force that is transmitted to the head"[3]
- "Classic presentation is impaired neurologic function with rapid onset and spontaneous resolution"[3]
- "Acute clinical signs and symptoms may be a result of neuropathological changes"[3]
- "Graded set of clinical signs and symptoms may or may not involve a loss of consciousness"[3]
- "Resolution of clinical and cognitive symptoms typically follows a sequential course"[3]

PATHOPHYSIOLOGY OF CONCUSSION

Most of the understanding of the pathophysiological processes of concussion are based on animal studies.[4] The widely agreed on pathophysiological process is the neurometabolic cascade and metabolic crisis.[1,2] These processes describe the pathophysiological process of concussion based on ionic shifts, impaired metabolism, and impaired neurotransmission.

The neurometabolic cascade is characterized by an initial depolarization of neuronal membranes.[4,5] An initial ion shift occurs when the biomechanical forces are applied to the brain and a large increase in excitatory amino acids, glutamate, release occurs.[1] This increase causes a potassium (K^+) as well as sodium (Na^+) and calcium (Ca^{2+}) efflux. The calcium ion–induced vasoconstriction reduces cerebral blood flow and glucose delivery with a resultant state of "metabolic depression," as the brain energy demand is not met by the vascular energy supply.[5] The neural and vascular tissue results in at first a hypermetabolic glycolytic state, as the neurons attempt to restore equilibrium.[2]

The metabolic crisis occurs when, in order to restore neuronal membrane potential, Na^+/K^+ pump work load increases. The Na^+/K^+ pumps require adenosine triphosphate (ATP) to create an equilibrium in the membrane potential.[4] The need for ATP also increases the demand for glucose metabolism. This increased need is present in a state of hypermetabolism when there is decreased cerebral blood flow, which creates a "metabolic mismatch" or "energy crisis."[4]

This complex cascade has also been shown to render neural tissue more susceptible to further injury, which may explain the rare, yet much publicized phenomenon of second-impact syndrome.[5] A second-impact injury occurs to the brain when the primary concussion has not resolved. This second impact increases intracranial blood volume, and there is a posttraumatic catecholamine release.[5] The brain is less able to respond adequately to the second injury and potentially leads to catastrophic cerebral edema.[5]

EVALUATION OF SPORTS-RELATED CONCUSSION

When evaluating a sports-related concussion, a thorough concussion examination should include a comprehensive history, neurologic examination, Sports Concussion Assessment Tool 5th edition (SCAT5), assessment of Glasgow Coma Scale, and cervical spine examination. Concussion history intake should also include a review of comorbidities along with previously sustained concussions. Neuroimaging in the acute setting of a concussion is often negative. However, the sideline and clinical examination may have some differences. A sport-related concussion is a diagnosis made by a well-trained medical professional in sports concussions, as there are no concrete tests or images that definitely diagnose sports-related concussion.

Sideline evaluations or screenings are challenging due to circumstances surrounding sporting events. Often there is an immediate need to assess the athlete quickly with sound medical decision-making to return-to-play or no return-to-play for the athlete. These screenings can include the SCAT5, a neurologic examination, a balance examination, visual assessment, and cervical spine examination, whereas they are not limited to only these evaluations.[6] The most important evaluation is to recognize concussion symptoms (headache, imbalance, loss of consciousness, whiplash, etc.) so that a decision of no return-to-play or return-to-play can be made to ensure the safety of the player. If a concussion is suspected, the athlete or player should be removed from sporting event until reevaluation can be completed.[3]

COMPREHENSIVE HISTORY

The comprehensive history begins with report of the mechanism of injury and intake of signs and symptoms that indicate concussion.[3] The SCAT5 for the athletes older than 12 years has 22 signs and symptoms graded on a 1 to 6 scale with 6 being the most severe:

SCAT5 signs and symptoms graded on a 1-6 scale: (for the athletes older than 12 y)	
• Headache	• "Don't feel right"
• "Pressure in head"	• Difficulty with memory or concentration
• Neck pain	• Fatigue or low energy
• Nausea or vomiting	• Confusion
• Balance problems	• Drowsiness
• Dizziness	• More emotional
• Balance problems	• Irritability
• Blurred vision	• Sadness
• Photophobia	• Nervous/anxious
• Phonophobia	• Trouble falling asleep
• Feeling slowed down	
• Feeling "like in a fog"	

These symptoms are gathered as initial injury baseline data in order to document the trend of signs and symptoms increasing or decreasing over the clinical course. The key to recording the trend of these signs and symptoms is adequate reporting from the patient and to limit the exposure to the SCAT5 when done serially. There is anecdotal and evidence-based research that athletes and patients will underreport in the hopes of being cleared to return to sport.[6,7]

The history also includes discussing the comorbidities for concussion, which is imperative. It is a long-held practice that 3 concussions in 1 calendar year is a red flag for not being able to provide medical clearance for return to sport regardless of age of the athlete. There is little or no evidence-based medicine on this long-held practice. However, there are data that support that once an athlete has sustained one concussion he/she is more susceptible to sustaining another concussion. As the number of concussions, in the concussion history, increases, so does the increased likelihood of sustaining additional concussions.[7] There are numerous factors that can contribute to the clinical course of a concussion, such as

- Number of symptoms
- Duration of symptoms greater than 4 weeks[3]
- History of previous concussion and details
- Past medical and family history of
  - Learning disabilities
  - Depression
  - Attention-deficit disorder/attention-deficit hyperactivity disorder
  - Sleep disorders
  - Migraines
  - Other psychiatric conditions

NEUROLOGIC EXAMINATION

On the sideline and in a clinical setting a neurologic examination should include, but not be limited to, cranial nerve testing, myotomes, dermatomes, and deep tendon reflexes. The neurologic examination should also include documentation of gait and balance. The gait can be screened initially with tandem gait balance. The SCAT5 provides further evaluation with the Modified Balance Error Scoring System.[8] The SCAT5 provides excellent instruction on how to conduct this examination and scoring for this important data point.[9]

NEUROIMAGING

Most sports-related concussions are an injury to the function of the brain; therefore, imaging is not necessary unless the neurologic examination clinically indicates a need for imaging.[3] Within the first 7 days of a concussion, a CT scan would be appropriate to order. After 7 days an MRI of the brain without contrast would be ordered. In the absence of a positive neurologic examination, advanced imaging is not indicated.

SPORTS CONCUSSION ASSESSMENT TOOL 5TH EDITION

The SCAT was developed by the Concussion In Sport Group (CISG) in 2004 for a guideline to assist in concussion evaluation. CISG then revised the SCAT in 2008, 2012, and 2016. The 2016 meeting lead the most recent SCAT5.[3] The SCAT5 was designed, for trained health care providers in SCAT5, to separate out sports-related concussion evaluation for child (5–12 years old) and adult (13 years old and older) athletes. However, this evaluation tool is not to be used exclusively for diagnosis of concussion.[8,9]

When administered efficiently, the SCAT5 should take approximately 10 minutes to test, which may require a noise-free environment. However, the SCAT5 does in fact have limitations toward athletes with disabilities and cultural and language differences.

Again, the results do not exclusively exist in the diagnosis of sports-related concussion.[8]

Both versions of the SCAT5 contain the red flag signs and symptoms to recognize and immediately seek a higher level of care.[8] These signs or symptoms include the following:

- Neck pain or tenderness
- Double vision
- Weakness or tingling/burning in arms or legs
- Severe or increasing headache
- Seizure or convulsion
- Loss of consciousness
- Deteriorating conscious state
- Vomiting
- Increasingly restless, agitated, or combative

GLASGOW COMA SCALE

Glasgow coma scale (GCS) is also used in both versions of the SCAT5. The GCS can be conducted serially in the setting of a deteriorating clinical presentation. The GCS consists of 3 categories that are rated on a 1 to 6 scale based on level of responsiveness: best eye, verbal, and motor response.[8,9]

CERVICAL SPINE EXAMINATION

A cervical spine examination is, also, imperative to document due to ascertaining a likelihood of a dual diagnosis of concussion and cervical spine (c-spine) injury. The c-spine injury must be prioritized over concussion signs/symptoms. It should be emphasized that the standard of practice, in a sideline or clinical setting, for an athlete who is not fully conscious or lucid is to assume there is a c-spine injury and follow all protocols to protect the c-spine.[8] A c-spine examination should include documenting presence or absence of c-spine point tenderness; pain or pain-free active range of movement in cervical flexion and extension; and lastly, documentation of c-spine myotomes bilaterally, which is imperative.[8]

MANAGEMENT OF SPORTS-RELATED CONCUSSION

According to the 5th International Conference on Concussion in Sport Berlin Guidelines from October 2016 (Berlin guidelines), there are 11 Rs when approaching the concussed patient and his/her management: recognize, remove, reevaluate, rest, rehabilitation, refer, recover, return to sports, reconsider, residual effect and sequelae, and risk reduction.[8] For the purpose of this article, the authors focus on school (return to learn), screen activity, sleep, social activity, and sports (return-to-play) with rest implemented in each area. With school and cognitive activities, it is important that there is a thoughtful process in return-to-learn yet custom tailored to the athlete's goal. Although return-to-sports will follow the Berlin guidelines.

RETURN-TO-SCHOOL GUIDELINES

The return-to-learn process is very individualized and may begin with a few days to a week of cognitive rest. On return to school, it may be necessary to start off part-time school or studying while working full-time (**Table 1**). For example, school participation does not need to focus on specific classes, but rather, let the patient choose the best

Table 1
Return-to-school guidelines

Mental Activity	Activity at Each Step	Goal of Each Step
1. Daily activities that do not give the child symptoms	Typical activities that are done during the day that do not increase symptoms (reading, screen time, etc) Start with 5–15 min and build up	Gradual return to typical activities
2. School Activities	Homework, reading, or other cognitive activities outside the classroom	Increase tolerance to cognitive work
3. Return to s chool part-time	Gradual introduction of school work. May need to start with partial school day or with increased breaks during the day	Increase the academic activities
4. Return to school full-time	Gradually progress school activities until a full day can be tolerated	Return to full academic activities and catch up on missed work

time of the day he/she could attend. The time of day of school could start off as 1 class or around 2 hours. After 3 days, they will increase his/her school time by 1 class or 2 hours. He/she will continue doing this, increasing class every 3 days until he/she reaches full-time school participation. The patient should work with their school to a less noisy area for classes such as physical education, band, choir, lunch, or any other classes that induce sound sensitivity symptoms.[3]

SCREEN ACTIVITY

In addition to discussing return-to-learn or school activities, addressing screen activity or computer usage is important during recovery.[3] In these current times, technology is used to communicate, learn, and set appointments and for entertainment. The athlete needs guidance on the usage of technology during the time surrounding cognitive rest from a concussion. Similar to return-to-learn and return-to-play, a slow progression back to screen activity is advised. The patient would benefit from resting by removing himself/herself from technology before symptoms emerge or worsen. At this time, there are no evidence-based guidelines to direct the usage of technology with sports-related concussions, specifically regarding the factors that surround technology, such as amount of time, resolution, light brightness, or size of screen.

SLEEP

There is some data that demonstrate sleep is disrupted with the onset of concussions. Athletes may either have increased or decreased sleep. There are also data for practicing good sleep hygiene guidance and decreasing screen time before bedtime.[10] When recovering from a sports-related concussion, the difference between rest and sleep should be discussed in great detail. Sleep may or may not be affected with concussions in which there is an increase of sleeping. As the clinical course progresses, there may be a trend of patients having a decrease in sleep, which can be contributed to not being as active. A recent study showed "good-quality sleep" improved concussion healing time, whereas poor-quality sleep increased healing time.[10]

SOCIAL ACTIVITY

Another factor in the management of sports-related concussion in the youth and adolescent population is social activity. The medical provider should recognize its importance and encourage the patient to engage in social activities in which these activities could be negotiated with the family. The athlete could attend practices and competitions contributing in what manner which the practitioner and/or coach allow him/her to be included in the team dynamics: record statistics, junior coach, or hand out water, etc.[11]

There are also school activities that would be appropriate to attend; however, it is important that the parents or guardian talk with the athlete about what are the expectations. For example, a loud musical concert is probably not best for recovering from a sports-related concussion. Instead spending time at a friends' house for a few hours would benefit the athlete's overall well-being. There should be an understanding that resting between or during activities would help allow the athlete to fully participate without flaring up symptoms.[11]

RETURN-TO-PLAY GUIDELINES

With regard to sports or physical activity, the data demonstrate that having the athlete do some level of movement is important.[3] If the patient is symptomatic, start off with either walking or stationary bike at low levels for short duration. The goal here is to get some movement. Most athletes are used to moving; this can assist with reducing the risk of depression. Much like cognitive activity, there will be an increase in physical activity in the absence or decrease of symptoms.[3] For example, if the athlete wants to start with 5 minutes of walking each day, he/she will do that for 3 days and increase by 3 to 5 minutes at a time. The goal would be to not increase or bring on postconcussion symptoms during the activity.

Once the trained medical provider has deemed it appropriate, a return-to-play guideline that follows the 6 steps described by Berlin consensus statement (refer to **Table 2**) can be used.[3] Before the return to play program, all patients must be in school full-time without symptoms such as headache, dizziness, blurred vision, and/or

Table 2
Return-to-play guidelines

Rehab Stage/Step	Functional Exercise	Objective
1. Symptom-limited activity	Daily activities that do not provoke symptoms	Gradual introduction of work/school activities
2. Light aerobic exercise	Walking, swimming, or stationary bike; no resistance training	Increase heart rate
3. Sport-specific exercise	Running drills; no head impact activities	Add movement
4. Noncontact training drills	Progression to more complex training drills; start progressive resistance training	Exercise, coordination, increasing thinking/cognitive load
5. *Full-contact practice*	*After medical clearance only; normal activity*	*Restores confidence and assesses functional skills by coaching staff*
6. Return to play	Normal game/competition	

pressure in head before starting the return-to-play program.[3] Each step will consist of physical activity that does not endorse symptoms during the activity or for a 24-hour period after the activity. Once the step has been completed without symptoms and resting from activity for 24 hours, the athlete can move to the next step 24 hours later. A written clearance letter to return to sports by an approved medical provider, per each state law, is required to return to full safe participation in the desired sport.[3]

OTHER CONSIDERATIONS

Over-the-counter or prescription medication has not proved to aid in healing or symptom control of a sports-related concussion.[3] With regard to routinely prescribed medications, it is important for the patient to continue all medications and not stop them unless instructed by their prescribing provider. It is important to recognize medications that may have a side effect of headaches or other concussion symptoms. The parent or guardian should contact the prescribing provider for further instructions on continued medication use during recovery from a sports-related concussion.

Although there has not been evidence-based research, many athletes may use home remedies to decrease symptoms. For example, it may be helpful to decrease headaches by going to a quiet room with no natural light, cold compresses, and warm showers. The use of these home remedies can be patient dependent.

REFERRALS

The Berlin consensus statement endorsed if symptoms persist for more than 10 to 14 days in adults or more than 4 weeks in children, a referral to a sports concussion specialist is warranted.[3] Sports-related concussions with persistent signs and symptoms can be overwhelming to treat by the primary care provider. Therefore, the patient is referred for a treatment by a multidisciplinary team that would include a sport concussion program with sports medicine providers, Certified Athletic Trainers, Sports Physical Therapist, Sports Neuropsychologist, and other closed head injury medical providers.[3]

RESOURCES

There are many resources for medical providers to access for assistance with sports-related concussion. Some resources emphasize management including Websites and Applications (apps). The resources may include information that aligns with the SCAT5 for child and adult and basic neurologic examination (refer to **Table 3** and **Box 1**).

Table 3 Concussion Website resources	
Control Center of Disease (CDC)	https://www.cdc.gov/headsup/index.html
American Academy of Neurology (AAN)	https://www.aan.com/Concussion
Concussion Legacy Foundation	https://concussionfoundation.org/
Sports Concussion Institute	http://concussiontreatment.com/
American Academy of Pediatrics (AAP)	https://www.aap.org/
National Athletic Trainer's Association (NATA)	https://www.nata.org/
American Academy of Family Practice (AAFP)	https://www.aafp.org/
Brain Injury Guidelines	https://braininjuryguidelines.org/ pediatricconcussion/

<table>
<tr><td>

Box 1
Concussion Applications (apps): iPhone and *Android compatible

*CDC HEADS UP Concussion and Helmet Safety

Concussion Tracker

*easySCAT

*Concussion Quick Check

*CSX

</td></tr>
</table>

SUMMARY

Sports-related concussions have been a current topic in the long-term wellness of all youth athletes in sport. Many articles have been written about evaluation and management of youth sports–related concussion. The 5th International Conference on Concussion in Sport Berlin Guidelines from October 2016 has been the sentinel beacon for guidelines used by many sports concussion providers.[3] This landmark article provides a comprehensive approach in sports-related concussion evaluation, management, and prevention in the sports-related concussion arena. The emphasis for sports-related concussion is to obtain a clear understanding of concussion evaluation, management of symptoms, and recognizing when to refer patients to sports concussion specialist.[3]

DISCLOSURE

The authors have nothing to disclose.

REFERENCES

1. Marar M, McIlvain NM, Fields SK, et al. Epidemiology of concussions among United States high school athletes in 20 sports. Am J Sports Med 2012;40(4): 747–55.
2. Lincoln AE, Caswell SV, Almquist JL, et al. Trends in concussion incidence in high school sports: a prospective 11-year study. Am J Sports Med 2011;39(5):958–63.
3. McCrory P, Meeuwisse WH, Dvorak J, et al. Consensus statement on concussion in sport: the 5th international conference on concussion in sport held in Berlin, October 2016. Br J Sports Med 2017;51(21):1557–8.
4. Giza CC, Hovda DA. The new neurometabolic cascade of concussion. Neurosurgery 2014;75(Suppl):S24–33.
5. Shrey DW, Griesbach GS, Giza CC. The pathophysiology of concussions in youth. Phys Med Rehabil Clin N Am 2011;22:577–602.
6. Patricios J, Fuller GW, Ellenbogen R, et al. What are the critical elements of sideline screening that can be used to establish the diagnosis of concussion? A systematic review. Br J Sports Med 2017;51(11):888–94.
7. Mahooti N. Sports-Related Concussion Acute Management and Chronic Postconcussive Issues. Child Adolesc Psychiatr Clin N Am 2018;27:93–108.
8. Echemendia RJ, Meeuwisse W, McCrory P, et al. The Sport Concussion Assessment Tooth 5th Edition (SCAT 5). Br J Sports Med 2017;51(21):848–50.
9. Davis GA, Purcell P, Schneider KJ, et al. The Child Sport Concussion Tool 5th Edition (Child SCAT 5). Br J Sports Med 2017;51(21):859–86.

10. Stewart N, Black L. Good Sleep Quality Encourages Better Recovery After Sport-Related Concussion. American Academy of Pediatrics. Available at: https://www.aap.org/en-us/about-the-aap/aap-press-room/pages/Good-Sleep-Quality-Encourages-Better-Recovery-After-Sport-Related-Concussion.aspx. Accessed November 2, 2018.
11. van Biljon A. Encouraging Your Child's Social Life After a Concussion Diagnosis. CognitiveX. Available at: https://www.cognitivefxusa.com/blog/encouraging-your-childs-social-life-after-a-concussion-diagnosis. Accessed February 22, 2019.

Pediatric Idiopathic Scoliosis Diagnosis and Management

Ana Maria G. Kolenko, PA-C, MPH[a], Jennifer M. Bauer, MD, MS[b],*

KEYWORDS

- Adolescent idiopathic scoliosis • Juvenile idiopathic scoliosis
- Infantile idiopathic scoliosis • Thoracolumbar bracing • Spinal fusion • Risser score
- Sanders score

KEY POINTS

- Idiopathic scoliosis is a diagnosis of exclusion in otherwise healthy patients and poses a risk of causing significant deformity.
- Scoliosis is diagnosed on radiographic images when there is a Cobb angle of 10° or greater.
- Bracing is the gold standard treatment in idiopathic scoliosis of the skeletally immature child.
- Primary care providers play a key role in identifying and appropriately referring patients with scoliosis to orthopedic specialists.

INTRODUCTION

Scoliosis is defined as a side-to-side or lateral curvature of the spine that is equal to or greater than 10°, but deformity exists in all 3 planes.[1] Scoliosis often is detected in the primary care setting and awareness is important, because it has the potential to cause severe musculoskeletal deformity. It can be associated with numerous etiologies, including the major categories of idiopathic, neuromuscular, congenital, and syndromic scoliosis. Thorough evaluation and examination are necessary to identify the cause for each patient's scoliosis. When no cause is identified, idiopathic scoliosis is diagnosed. Although pediatric scoliosis may develop from an array of underlying disorders, more than 80% of children diagnosed with scoliosis have idiopathic scoliosis.[1]

[a] Orthopedics and Sports Medicine, Seattle Children's Hospital, 4800 Sand Point Way Northeast, M/S OA.9.120, Seattle, WA 98105, USA; [b] Seattle Children's Hospital, University of Washington Orthopedics and Sports Medicine, 4800 Sand Point Way Northeast, M/S OA.9.120, Seattle, WA 98105, USA
* Corresponding author.
E-mail address: Jennifer.bauer@seattlechildrens.org

Physician Assist Clin 5 (2020) 441–453
https://doi.org/10.1016/j.cpha.2020.06.001
physicianassistant.theclinics.com

Scoliosis affects all ages and is subdivided into 3 age groups: infantile scoliosis diagnosed between 0 and 3 years of age, juvenile scoliosis between 4 and 10 years of age, and, the largest group, adolescent scoliosis diagnosed over 10 years of age.[2] The age of onset is important because scoliotic deformity progresses in accordance with the amount of remaining skeletal growth. Although risk of progression is greatest with the adolescent growth spurt, the younger the child the higher the likelihood for continued curve progression given the overall longer period of height growth. Most curves cause only a mild clinical deformity of the trunk; however, when severe, scoliosis has the potential to become markedly disfiguring causing significant cardiopulmonary compromise. Irrespective of the curve magnitude, scoliosis can lead to a decreased quality of life and accurate diagnosis and management are important for appropriate patient care. This review focuses on idiopathic scoliosis across all age groups and includes the critical diagnosis and management principles to better guide practitioners' care.

IDIOPATHIC SCOLIOSIS

Idiopathic scoliosis is a musculoskeletal disorder from unknown etiology affecting all age groups but occurring most commonly in adolescence. Idiopathic scoliosis is a diagnosis of exclusion requiring thorough evaluation for possible underlying disorders.[2] Genetic, metabolic, mechanical, and hormonal causes have been suggested, but no definitive etiology has yet been determined.[3] The rate of deformity progression is directly correlated with spinal growth and skeletal immaturity. For this reason, younger age of onset is associated with a higher risk of curve progression.[4] In the general population, approximately 2% to 3% of children under the age of 16 have a spinal curvature greater than or equal to 10°.[5] An even smaller percentage progress to needing some type of medical intervention.

Most patients diagnosed with idiopathic scoliosis have no symptoms and are identified during their routine wellness examination. Often the presence of a truncal shift or uneven shoulders clues providers into a possible underlying spinal curvature.[6] For this reason, astute clinical awareness and thorough examination are critical to diagnosis. If scoliosis goes undetected, especially in the infantile and juvenile groups, curves may reach over 70° in magnitude. A curvature of this size compromises patients' health and is correlated with an increased risk of cardiovascular and pulmonary compromise.[4,7]

History

Visits should be detailed and include a past medical and family history. A systematic history can exclude underlying etiologies potentially causing or contributing to nonidiopathic scoliosis, which may need a different treatment or work-up than idiopathic cases. When collecting medical history, inquire whether others in the family have scoliosis because there is a hereditary association. When compared with the general population, a patient with an affected parent is 3 times more likely to develop scoliosis.[6] This rate increases to 7 times as likely with an affected sibling. Patients with a family history of syndromic, genetic, or neuromuscular disorders may need additional evaluation for such inherited conditions. For example, connective tissue disorders, such as Marfan syndrome and Ehlers-Danlos syndrome, are associated with development of scoliosis. History of delayed milestones also may signal that there is a potential underling neuromuscular disorder affecting growth and development. The past surgical history is important because thoracogenic scoliosis occurs at larger rates in children with previous thoracotomies.[6]

When recording a patient's history, also inquire about current symptoms and include a targeted review of systems. Although idiopathic scoliosis often is asymptomatic, studies have shown that upwards of 23% of children with idiopathic scoliosis experience back pain.[8] In those with back pain, 9% subsequently are found to have an underling pathology. In some, it may not be pain but physical appearance that bothers them most. Children, in particular adolescents, may notice asymmetry in their shoulders or waist. Commonly parents may notice clothing falling differently on their child's back.

Intraspinal pathologies sometimes are associated with scoliosis or are the driving factors behind the deformity. Signs and symptoms may be subtle and, when present with scoliosis, a detailed review of systems can detect cases of Chiari malformations, tethered cords, and syringomyelias. These intraspinal pathologies may present as gait disturbances or asymmetric reflexes. Therefore, a neurologic history inquiring about daily activities, such as walking and running, and bladder or bowel incontinence should be included. Base of the skull headaches with activity or Valsalva maneuvers although rare, when present with scoliosis may signify a Chiari malformation. Asymmetric foot arches and a progressive scoliosis may indicate a tethered cord.

For female patients, onset of menses is important when considering skeletal maturity. Menarche onset is a predictor for time of rapid growth, slows over a 2-year period thereafter.[9] Scoliosis progresses most rapidly during peak growth velocity, which can be predicted with serial height measurements, menarche, secondary signs of puberty, a growth chart, and closure of the triradiate cartilage on radiographs.[9]

Clinical Examination

Physical examination of the spine as well as the entire musculoskeletal and neurologic system is imperative. Boys should be evaluated in shorts and girls in shorts and bra for proper evaluation. Begin with a general examination of the patient, evaluating strength and range of motion of the bilateral upper and lower extremities. Assess for underlying hypotonia or hypertonia suggesting a neuromuscular scoliosis. Ensure there is no asymmetric muscle tone of the lower extremities or presence of a unilateral cavovarus foot or toe clawing, which can be associated with a tethered cord. A detailed neurologic examination includes assessment of reflexes and sensory function of the upper and lower extremities, and nerve tension examinations, such as a straight leg raise. Reflexes examined should include abdominal, patellar, Achilles, and evaluation for clonus. Abdominal reflex is performed by gently stroking the abdomen on either side of the umbilicus, which triggers a contraction of the abdominal muscles toward the source of stimulation. An asymmetric contraction response, in conjunction with other abnormal clinical signs, should trigger further work-up to rule out an intraspinal disorder. It is important also to observe a patient's gait; a limp or truncal shift may signify a leg length discrepancy masquerading as postural scoliosis. If present, level the pelvis with the appropriate under-shoe lift prior to spine examination.

When examining the spine, start with general inspection of posture from the front, back, and sides. Scoliosis often causes asymmetric shoulder height, chest wall rotational deformity, and rib prominences as well as lumbar back prominences from curves in the lower back. Children with larger habitus may be difficult to examine and asymmetric waist folds can clue clinicians into an underlying scoliosis. Confirm the pelvis is level by palpating the lateral iliac crests to ensure that there is no pelvic obliquity. Assess the patient's skin because abnormalities, such as café au lait spots and axillary freckles, are associated with neurofibromatosis, another cause of neuromuscular scoliosis. Midline abnormalities, including patches of hair, skin pits, or dimples, can signify underlying spinal dysraphism, which may imply congenital defects of the spinal cord and vertebrae.[2] Tenderness to palpation is not common; however, children with significant pain may have underlying pathology that warrants further imaging.[2] When tenderness is present and related to scoliosis, it may be from fatigue in the paraspinal muscles at the convex apex of large curves or rhomboids in the thoracic spine. Low midline back pain or tenderness may indicate an underlying spondylolysis or spondylolisthesis, unrelated to the scoliosis.[2]

Most importantly, clinicians should feel confident in preforming an Adams forward bend test (**Fig. 1**). Test was first described in 1865 by William Adams and has become the mainstay for clinical examination of vertebral body rotation associated with scoliosis.[10] Because scoliosis has deformity in all 3 planes, a typical coronal curvature is associated with axial rotation, which causes the rib cage to twist along with the rotated spine. This gives the appearance of a prominence on the convex side of the curve and is more easily visible when bending forward. This test should be performed with the patient bending forward at the waist while maintaining straight knees, with legs and head loosely hanging down toward the floor.[2] The provider should then examine the back to look for presence of thoracic or lumbar prominence asymmetry. Clinical evidence of asymmetry to the thoracic and lumbar spines warrants further evaluation with radiography. This asymmetry can be quantified using a scoliometer, which is similar to a level laid horizontally along the back while in the forward bend position. A scoliometer reading of 5 often correlates to a Cobb angle of greater than 20°.[11] Although useful for detection, there is a large degree of user variability with this tool, and radiographs are preferred for continued curve monitoring.[11]

Diagnosis

Radiographic imaging is the gold standard for diagnosing scoliosis. Standing posterior-anterior (PA) and lateral radiographs should be obtained when there is

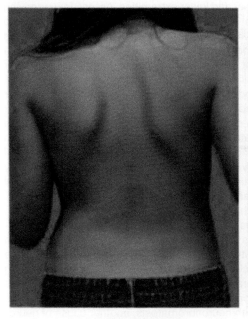 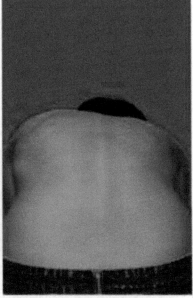

Standing   Forward bend test

Fig. 1. Adams forward bend test.

clinical suspicion. A standing film provides the most reliable curve measurement and takes into account gravitational effects on the spine. Seated upright films are acceptable if a patient is unable to stand. In the presence of a leg length discrepancy, a block under the shortened leg should be used to compensate for the difference in limb height. If a scoliometer was used during examination, a reading of 5° or greater should prompt further evaluation with imaging.

A normal radiograph without the presence of any curve can assure the patient and family that scoliosis is not present. Curves under 10° are consistent with spinal asymmetry, which is not associated with the development of scoliosis. The presence of a curve greater than 10° is diagnostic for scoliosis. Curves on radiograph are assessed with the use of the Cobb angle technique. The endplate of the most tilted vertebrae at the top and bottom of the curve is marked and a right angle line is drawn down from the top endplate line and up from the bottom endplate line. The angle created by the intersecting right angle lines indicates the Cobb angle (**Fig. 2**).[2]

Subsequently, assess the general radiographic appearance of the curve. Scoliotic curves assume a variety of curve patterns; however, adolescent idiopathic scoliosis most commonly presents as an S-shaped curve. Classically the proximal curve has a right thoracic apex and the distal curve a left lumbar apex, and a less obvious third left proximal thoracic curve occasionally can be measured. Sometimes the appearance is of a sole thoracic or lumbar curve. Curves also should have a notable amount vertebral body rotation, which is greatest at the apex (**Fig. 3**); if not, the curve may be from the child positioning the spine away from a painful stimuli and not from scoliosis. Vertebrae also should be assessed for the presence of a congenital deformity, such as triangular hemivertebra, instead of block-shaped bone or vertebrae that appear fused

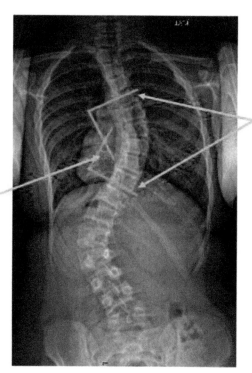

Line parallel to the most tilted proximal and distal vertebrae

Angle indicator: This is the Cobb angle

Fig. 2. Cobb angle measurement technique.

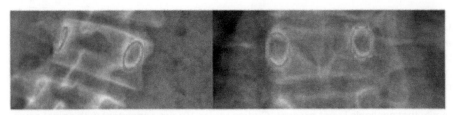

| Asymmetrical pedicles with vertebral body rotation | Symmetrical pedicles without vertebral body rotation |

Fig. 3. Vertebral body rotation in can be appreciated by the amount of pedicle (*circles*) asymmetry.

(**Fig. 4**). The presence of these congenital abnormalities makes the diagnosis a congenital scoliosis.

Understanding the properties of a typical idiopathic curve is critical for identifying scoliotic curves that require additional imaging. Curves that lack vertebral body rotation, contain congenital anomalies, have left thoracic or right lumbar apexes, or are sweeping C-shaped may be driven by an underlying pathology. In these patients, a total spine magnetic resonance image (MRI) without contrast is recommended.[12] Patients with very rapid progression, a curve over 20° before the age of 10, significant pain, or abnormal physical examinations also should be referred for an MRI, given the risk of intraspinal pathology. When ordering an MRI for these reasons, consider and counsel the family on the possible presence of a syrinx, Chiari malformation, tethered cord, or other intraspinal pathology (**Fig. 5**). If there is an abnormal MRI or abnormal physical examination and history, the patient does not have idiopathic scoliosis.

An important part of idiopathic scoliosis management is also assessing for skeletal and spinal growth, important predictors for curve progression. Providers should

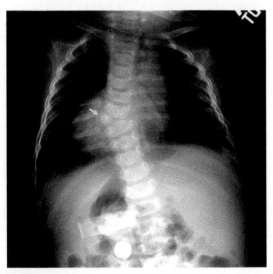

Fig. 4. Hemivertebrae (*arrow*) causing congenital scoliosis.

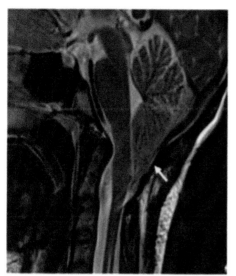 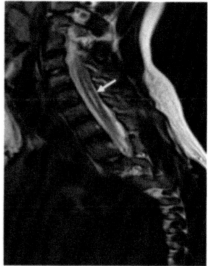

Chiari malformation. Herniation of the cerebellum through the foramen magnum into the spinal canal.

Syrinx. Dilated fluid-filled central canal of the spinal cord.

Fig. 5. Neural axis abnormalities in patients with scoliosis.

appreciate the different approaches to assessing skeletal maturity and how they apply to scoliosis. There are several radiographic ways to assess maturity; the most common is the Risser score, but there is low inter-rater reliability.[6] This score assesses the iliac crest apophysis ossification, which, when fused to the ilium, correlates with the completion of growth and is scored on a 0 to 5 continuum (**Fig. 6**). Risser score should be appreciated on PA radiographs of the pelvis and often is included within spine films. Most rapid skeletal growth occurs before Risser stage 1 is appreciated on imaging just after the triradiate pelvic cartilage closes.[6] Patients who are Risser stage 0 are subdivided into 2 groups: with or without closure of the triradiate cartilage.

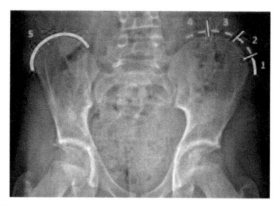

Fig. 6. Risser score.

Patients who are Risser stage 0 with open triradiate cartilages are at significant risk for progression because they have not yet entered their peak growth velocity. A more reliable method for assessing spinal growth recently was adopted, known as the Sanders score. This assessment uses a PA film of the hand, also known as a bone age, and divides skeletal growth into 8 stages. Stage 1 correlates with slow juvenile growth, usually between 8 years and 10 years of age whereas stage 8 correlates with skeletal maturity, usually ages 17 years to 19 years old. This approach is beneficial because it allows providers to identify children as they enter their rapid stage of growth, which is Sanders stage 3, and when spinal growth has completed at Sanders stage 7.[13] Research is ongoing for alternative measurements with higher interobserver reliability than Risser and Sanders scores, which include assessing the apophysis of the thumb or proximal humerus.

Management

Once a diagnosis of idiopathic scoliosis is made, appropriate treatment for patient's age should commence. Although diagnostic guidelines are similar for all age groups, treatment and natural history vary. Most skeletally immature patients with curves 20° to 25° or greater should start treatment and be referred to an orthopedic provider for continued management.

ADOLESCENT IDIOPATHIC SCOLIOSIS

Adolescent idiopathic scoliosis makes up the largest group of scoliosis cases, with 2% to 3% of the adolescent population being affected.[5] Approximately 5% to 10% of those affected go on to need bracing and another 0.1% progress to need surgical management.[1,6,14] The goal of treatment should be to prevent or halt curve progression. Treatment generally falls into 3 categories: observation, bracing, and surgery. Curves that are greater than 10° but less than 20° should have continued observation with a 1-view PA radiograph every 6 months to 9 months. A majority of adolescent curves stay below 20°. Consider curves between 20° and 40° for bracing and refer curves over 40° to an orthopedic surgeon for surgical discussion.

In large patient studies, once children reach skeletal maturity, curves under 35° remain relatively stable. A majority of curves greater than 50° continue to progress even after skeletal maturity by an average of 1° a year and, therefore, can reach much larger sizes if untreated into adulthood.[15] Large curves may cause back pain or significant cosmetic deformity and, more importantly, contribute to cardiac and pulmonary compromise.[6] Identifying which patients have curves that will progress is essential for initiating the appropriate treatment.

Bracing

The cornerstone of nonoperative scoliosis treatment is bracing. The Bracing in Adolescent Idiopathic Scoliosis Trial (BRAIST) unwaveringly supported the use of bracing to control curve progression and decrease the likelihood of surgical intervention.[16] The BRAIST study found that 52% of children without bracing went on to develop curves requiring surgery compared with 28% who were treated with bracing, and less so with higher brace-wear compliance. Knowing when to start, which brace to use, and for how long to use it can be daunting for providers new to scoliosis management. The fundamental recommendation is that bracing should be initiated in skeletally immature children (Risser stages 0–2) when a curve reaches 20° to 25°.[16,17] There are insufficient data to use Sanders staging for brace initiation; rather, its principles are best applied when assessing risk of progression and discontinuation of bracing.

Greatest success is seen when patients are started in a brace between 20° and 29° although larger curves should still be offered bracing. Curves greater than 50° are not routinely offered bracing because these are likely to progress throughout life whenever the brace is discontinued. It is important educate patients and families that bracing does not improve scoliosis but rather reduces the risk of progression and, therefore, surgical indication.

There are several types of full-time and nighttime spinal braces, most with similar efficacy, but with differing styles and corrective mechanical principles. The most common full-time brace is the thoracolumbar sacral orthosis, which includes the Boston and Wilmington brace styles. Nighttime orthoses include the Providence and Charleston braces. These nighttime braces provide an alternative to patients who are unlikely to be compliant with full-time bracing and have curves below 30°, but recent research suggests they may be efficacious in larger curves. Controversy continues over whether nighttime braces are inferior to full-time underarm orthosis; the authors prefer a full-time underarm brace when possible. Patients should obtain an in-brace PA radiograph after receiving their brace to determine effectiveness. Goal correction is at least 50% while in brace for full-time braces and greater than 75% for nighttime braces.[6]

Full-time underarm braces should be worn 18 hours daily because greater wear time is associated with less progression. Studies have shown that when patients wear their braces for at least 18 hours daily, there is a 90% to 93% success rate compared with a 42% success rate with 0 to 6 hours daily.[17] Success is defined as reaching skeletal maturity with a curve less than 50°. Studies also have shown lower success rates in a majority of patients who are Risser stage 0 with open triradiates at the time of initiating brace treatment.[16] Further research is needed, however, to understand whether bracing may at least delay the timing of surgical intervention. Alternatively, children who are Risser stage 2 and adhere to bracing rarely progress to needing surgery.[16]

After initiating bracing, a PA radiograph out of brace for up to a day prior can be obtained every 6 months to 9 months. These visits are important for monitoring progression. Imaging any more frequently has little added benefit and higher lifetime radiation exposure. Discontinue bracing when children either are skeletally mature or need surgical intervention. Spinal skeletal maturity is reached at Sanders stage 7. For girls, this is approximately 2 years after the onset of menarche. For both boys and girls, providers should also take into account plateau in height. If a patient has reached radiographic skeletal maturity but has continued to grow in height, bracing should be continued until height has plateaued.

Despite recommendations, many patients understandably resist bracing. It is important to have an honest discussion with the family and patient on when to start bracing and realistic wear time. Consider social factors, which play a large role into compliance. Male patients have more difficulty with brace compliance perhaps because of their body habitus or longer brace wear duration given their older age for reaching skeletal maturity compared with female patients.[6]

Surgery

Children who have curves approaching 50° should be referred to an orthopedic surgeon for consultation. The goals of surgical treatment include preventing curve progression while obtaining spinal correction, realignment, and multilevel fusion. Corrective surgeries most frequently follow a posterior approach, but anterior and a combination of anterior and posterior surgery are dependent on surgeon preference and curve type. Current techniques aim to either fuse the spine or modulate growth. Both posterior and anterior spinal fusions use a combination of implants to provide surgical correction and result in 15% to 48% Cobb angle improvement on the coronal plane (**Fig. 7**).[6] Growth modulation is a newer surgical technique that uses an anterior approach without fusion to realign the spine in skeletally immature children with a flexible tether, so as not to fuse the spine and retain motion. The risks and complications of surgery can be serious and the decision to pursue surgery should be a thoughtful and well-educated discussion.

EARLY-ONSET SCOLIOSIS

Idiopathic scoliosis also affects children below the age of 10 and is associated with more severe deformities and additional treatment approaches. Much of the prior discussion in the adolescent scoliosis group applies here; however, there are some notable differences to consider. Within this age group, there is further division into juvenile and infantile scoliosis.

Juvenile Scoliosis

Juvenile idiopathic scoliosis affects children between 4 years and 10 years of age and makes up approximately 15% of all idiopathic scoliosis cases.[18] When evaluating this patient population, it is important to know that there is a 18% to 25% incidence of

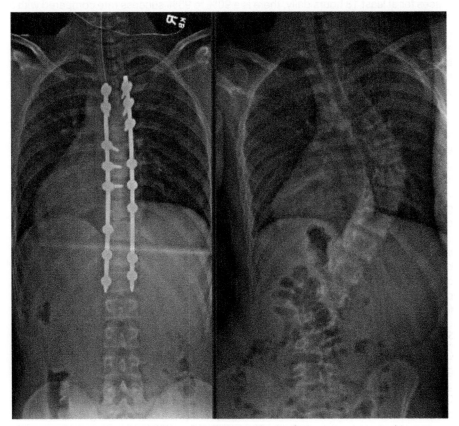

Fig. 7. Curve correction in adolescent idiopathic scoliosis after a posterior spinal instrumentation and fusion (*Left* - post-operative, *Right* - pre-operative.).

neural axis abnormalities, significantly higher than in the adolescent group. Such abnormalities include syringomyelia, Chiari malformation, and tethered cord, as discussed previously.[18] Given the young age of onset, there also is a higher risk of progression compared with adolescents. Approximately 70% of cases require treatment and upwards of 50% of cases progress to surgery. The bracing guidelines, discussed previously, apply to this population; however, corrective casting often is used as an alternative treatment in those under the age of 5.

Surgery is recommended once curves progress to 50° or greater. The goal at this age, however, is no longer a spinal fusion but rather growth-friendly techniques. These approaches maximize thoracic growth, ideally allowing for optimal cardiopulmonary development in the growing child, but treatment ends in a spinal fusion once appropriate thoracic height has been reached. Approaches include distraction-based systems, such as traditional growing rods, magnetically controlled growing rods, and vertically expandable prosthetic titanium rib; compression-based systems; and guided growth techniques, including the Shilla method and Luqué trolley (**Fig. 8**).[19] Spinal fusions generally are avoided at this age because there is strong evidence to show that an early fusion contributes to significant pulmonary compromise and severe spinal deformity.

Infantile Scoliosis

Infantile scoliosis is diagnosed in patients between 0 and 3 years of age and makes up 0.5% of all scoliosis cases.[6] It is estimated that 90% of these curves are left thoracic facing and, unlike adolescent scoliosis, upwards of 90% spontaneously resolve.[6] In this age group, the rib vertebral angle difference (RVAD) is an important measurement, used in conjunction with the Cobb angle, to predict progression. When curves are

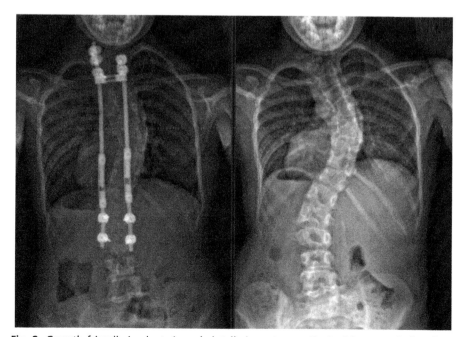

Fig. 8. Growth-friendly implants in a skeletally immature patient with congenital scoliosis (*Left* - post-operative, *Right* - pre-operative.).

greater than 20° and there is an RVAD over 20° on initial radiograph, they are less likely to resolve and warrant medical intervention.[18] The treatment of choice for this age group is serial derotational casting with Mehta technique. This casting technique improves thoracic and lumbar curves through the use of a derotation maneuver that helps straighten the spine and maintain alignment while casted. These casts are done under the supervision of a skilled orthopedist and applied every 3 months to 4 months with periodic imaging. Curves that are prone to resolution typically do so within a mean of 5 casting cycles.[20] Surgery largely is avoided in this age group.

DISCLOSURE

The author has nothing to disclose.

REFERENCES

1. Scoliosis Research Society. Scoliosis. Available at: https://www.srs.org/patients-and-families/conditions-and-treatments/parents/scoliosis. Accessed November 23, 2019.
2. Altaf F, Gibson A, Dannawi Z, et al. Adolescent idiopathic scolisosis. BMJ 2013; 346:1–7.
3. Asher M, Burton D. Adolescent idiopathic scoliosis: natural history and long term treatment effects. Scoliosis 2006;1:2.
4. Nachemson A. A long term follow-up study of non-treated scoliosis. Acta Orthop Scand 1968;39:466–76.
5. Weinstein S. The natural history of adolescent idiopathic scoliosis. J Pediatr Orthop 2019;39:S44–6.
6. Newton P, Yaszay B, Wenger D. Adolescent idiopathic scoliosis. In: Weinstein S, Flynn J, editors. Lovell & Winter's pediatric orthopedics. 7th edition. Philadelphia: Wolters Kluwer Health; 2014. p. 629–89.
7. Pehrsson K, Larsson S, Oden A, et al. Long-term followup of patients with untreated scoliosis: A study of mortality, causes of death, and symptoms. Spine 1992;17:1091–6.
8. Sanders J, Browne R, Cooney T, et al. Correlates of the peak height velocity in girls withidiopathic scoliosis. Spine 2006;31:2289–95.
9. Lonstein JE, Carlson JM. The prediction of curve progression in untreated idiopathic scoliosis during growth. J Bone Joint Surg 1984;66:1061–107.
10. Fairbank MJ. Historical perspective: William Adams, the forward bending test, and the spine of Gideon Algernon. Spine 2004;29:1953–5.
11. Cote P, Krietz BG, Cassidy JD, et al. A study of the diagnostic accuracy and reliability of the Scoliometer and Adam's forward bend test. Spine 1998;23(7): 796–802.
12. Barnes PD, Brody JD, Jaramillo D, et al. Atypical idiopathic scoliosis: MR imaging evaluation. Radiology 1993;186:247–53.
13. Sanders JO, Khoury JG, Kishan S, et al. Predicting scoliosis progression from skeletal maturity: a simplified classification during adolescence. J Bone Joint Surg Am 2008;90(3):540–53.
14. Tambe AD, Panikkar SJ, Millner PA, et al. Current concepts in the surgical management of adolescent idiopathic scoliosis. Bone Joint J 2018;100-B(4):415–24.
15. Weinstein SL, Ponseti IV. Curve progression in idiopathic scoliosis. J Bone Joint Surg Am 1983;65:447–55.

16. Karol LA, Virostek D, Felton K, et al. The effect of the risser stage on bracing outcome in adolescent idiopathic scoliosis. J Bone Joint Surg Am 2016;98(15): 1253–9.
17. Weinstein SL, Dolan LA, Wright JG, et al. Effects of bracing in adolescents with idiopathic scoliosis. N Engl J Med 2013;269:1512–21.
18. Orthbullets. Souder C. Juvenile Idiopathic Scoliosis. Available at: https://www.orthobullets.com/spine/2054/juvenile-idiopathic-scoliosisEOS1. Accessed November 20 2019.
19. Skaggs DL, Akbarnia BA, Flynn JM, et al. A classification of growth friendly spine implants. J Pediatr Orthop 2014;34:260–74.
20. Ramirez N, Johnston CE, Browne RH. The prevalence of back pain in children who have idiopathic scoliosis. J Bone Joint Surg Am 1997;79:364–8.

Pediatric Upper Extremity Trauma

Douglas S. Dedo, PA-C, MCHS

KEYWORDS

- Finger injuries • Trigger thumb • Clinodactyly • Ganglion cyst • Scaphoid fracture
- Radius and ulna forearm fractures

KEY POINTS

- Use a long arm cast in very young children to protect fractures from the fingertips to the elbow so that it does not slide off the arm.
- Use a soft cast instead of fiberglass material on young children to avoid the need for a noisy cast saw to remove it.
- Use chromic gut sutures in young children to avoid the need to have them return for a scary suture removal.
- When there is wrist pain from a fall, check the anatomic snuffbox for a scaphoid fracture.
- Look for a dislocation at the wrist with a distal radius fracture and at the elbow with a proximal ulna fracture.

INTRODUCTION

A normal aspect of being a child involves frequent falls. Young bones tend to be flexible and absorb a lot of impact well. However, there is a limit to the force children's bones can take before they are broken. Fifty percent of all pediatric fractures involve the upper extremities.[1] The following sections review common traumatic injuries to the hand and forearm and how best to treat them.

FINGER CRUSH INJURIES (TUFT FRACTURES, SEYMOUR FRACTURES, AND MALLET FINGERS)

Crushing injuries to the tip of a finger are common in children. This can happen when their finger is caught in a car door or when something heavy like a brick falls on their finger. The fingernail may be damaged, the soft tissue from the tip of the finger may be avulsed, and the bone may be broken (**Fig. 1**). Ketamine sedation or a digital block can make repairing this injury more comfortable for the child necessitating a visit to the emergency department.

There is a type of fracture, called a Seymour fracture, that occurs in the segment of the finger most distant from the body, the distal phalanx, which has a high risk of infection.

Orthopedics and Sports Medicine, Seattle Children's Hospital, 4800 Sand Point Way NE, Seattle, WA 98105, USA
E-mail address: Douglas.Dedo@seattlechildrens.org

Physician Assist Clin 5 (2020) 455–476
https://doi.org/10.1016/j.cpha.2020.06.005
2405-7991/20/© 2020 Elsevier Inc. All rights reserved.

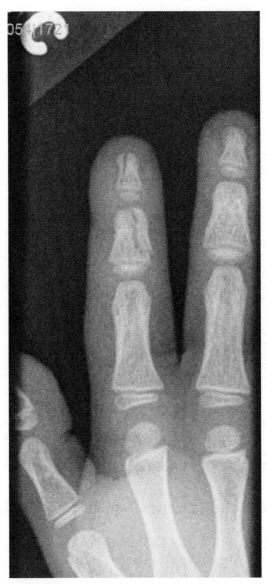

Fig. 1. Crush injuries sometimes cause longitudinal fracture lines as can be seen in the distal and middle phalanges of this index finger.

This is often caused by a crush injury such as when a finger gets slammed in a door. A Seymour fracture is a combination of a distal phalanx that is broken at the base, often through the growth plate (physis), combined with a finger nailbed injury (**Fig. 2**). If soft tissue (typically the germinal matrix of the nail) is caught in the fracture site, this should be treated in the emergency department. The severity of this fracture is often missed. A Seymour fracture is an open fracture and requires an antibiotic, such as cephalexin, for 7 to 10 days to prevent soft tissue infection and osteomyelitis, a bone infection.[2]

If there is an avulsed fingertip, suture it back in place to create a biologic dressing (**Fig. 3 and 4**). Even if the damaged portion does not survive, it will provide great

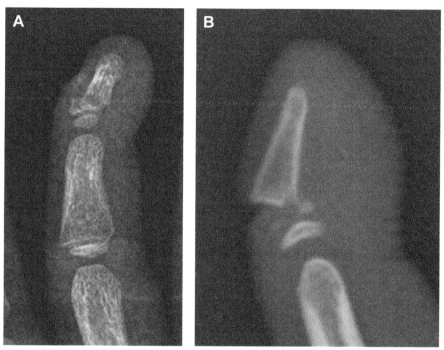

Fig. 2. (*A*) This is an example of a Seymour fracture, which is a combination of a displaced fracture at the base of the distal phalanx and disruption to the nailbed. (*B*) This is another example of a Seymour fracture with a combination of a displaced fracture at the base of the distal phalanx at the growth plate and disruption to the nailbed. Seymour fractures are open fractures with a high risk of infection.

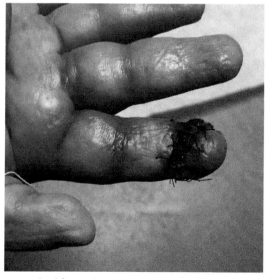

Fig. 3. Reattaching an avulsed fingertip creates a great biologic dressing. Unfortunately this provider used nylon sutures, so the child will need to return for suture removal.

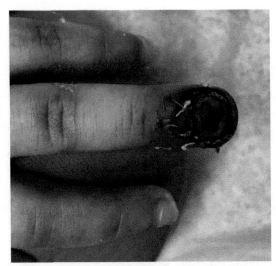

Fig. 4. Repair nailbed lacerations and secure the fingernail or a foil proxy under the epony-chial nail fold with 6-0 chromic gut (sutures that dissolve).

protection while the body heals the underlying tissue that has a good blood supply. If bone is exposed, this should be treated as an open fracture with antibiotics.

If suturing is required, use 6-0 chromic gut so that the sutures will dissolve. Do not use Fast Absorbing chromic gut; this is only effective for 5 to 7 days, and these wounds need to be secured for 10 to 14 days, which regular chromic gut provides. Removing nondissolvable sutures, like nylon or Prolene, from a young child's hand can be a scary experience for the child, parent, and provider.

To provide the best opportunity for a fingernail to grow out properly if the germinal ma-trix is not damaged, suture the fingernail in place so that it sits under the eponychial fold (**Fig. 4**). If the fingernail is too badly damaged or lost during the traumatic event (**Fig. 5**), use the foil packaging from the chromic gut suture to fabricate an artificial fingernail and suture this under the eponychial fold. This prevents the fold from scaring down, which blocks the new nail, created at the germinal matrix, from progressing past this firm tissue.

The dressing for a crush injury can start with petroleum gauze, such as Xeroform, over the damaged tissue. This provides an occlusive dressing that does not stick to

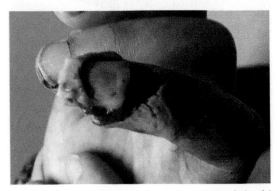

Fig. 5. The damage to this fingernail germinal matrix may result in this nail not growing back.

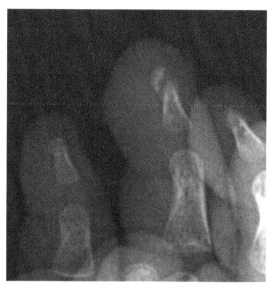

Fig. 6. A tuft fracture at the distal end of the distal phalanx.

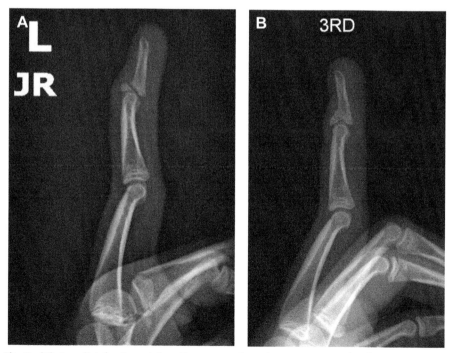

Fig. 7. (*A*) A mallet fracture deformity occurs when the extensor tendon becomes disconnected from the dorsal base of the distal phalanx sometimes causing an avulsion fracture. (*B*) After 6 weeks of wearing an extension splint, the bone fragment has become reattached with the distal phalanx, making a straight finger possible again.

the finger and reduces the risk of infection. Another characteristic of this type of gauze is that it can stay on a wound for weeks. A small roll of Kerlix can be placed in the palm for comfort. Cover the finger and hand with soft padding. Then apply a mitten cast over this dressing to help keep the injured finger clean and protected for 3 weeks. In very young children who are frightened by loud noises, use soft casting tape that can be unwound instead of the fiberglass material that requires a noisy cast saw for removal.

Fractures that occur at the neck of the segment of the finger most distant from the body, the distal phalanx, are called tuft fractures (**Fig. 6**). Depending on the age of the patient, a mitten cast, aluminum splint, or buddy taping can be utilized depending on the amount of protection needed to match the activity level and maturity of the child. Buddy taping involves applying half inch cloth tape on either side of the proximal inter-phalangeal (PIP) joints of 2 adjacent fingers. The tape should be worn around the clock and replaced after it has become wet, such as after bathing.

Fractures that occur at the base of the distal phalanx on the dorsum, or posterior side, of the bone can result in a mallet finger where the patient is unable to fully extend the tip of their finger (**Fig. 7**A). The shape made by the fingertip hanging down looks like a type of hammer called a mallet. This injury is commonly caused by something like a ball hitting the fingernail and forcing the fingertip down further than the extensor tendon can stretch causing the tendon to pull off a piece of the bone at the base of the distal phalanx. To treat this type of fracture, the finger is placed in an extension splint which holds the distal interphalangeal (DIP) joint firmly in extension nonstop for 6 weeks. It is ideal if there are two splints so that a dry one can be applied immediately after bathing. After the finger is no longer going to get wet, the splint is removed while maintaining pressure on the finger pad until it can be placed in a new dry extension splint. This can be done by holding one's finger in extension by pressing down on a

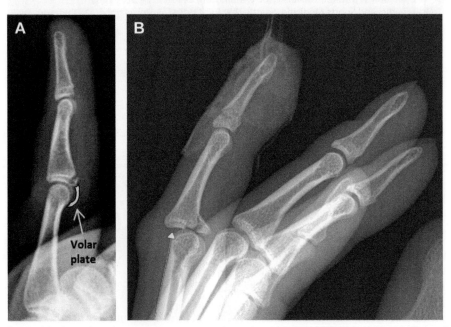

Fig. 8. (A) The volar plate is a ligament on the palm side that attaches to the middle and proximal phalanges. Hyperextension at this joint can cause an avulsion fracture at the base of the middle phalanx. (B) This middle phalanx with a volar plate injury is also subluxed and will require surgery. Note how the dorsal edges of the middle and proximal phalanges do not line up at the yellow arrow.

counter or on one's thigh. A Stack (or Stax) splint that securely holds the finger or a custom dorsal extension splint made by an occupational therapist is appropriate depending on which fits best and is most comfortable. If radiograph imaging at six weeks does not show a clear bony bridge between the fragment and the rest of the distal phalanx (**Fig. 7**B), an extension splint should be worn for another 6 weeks. In some cases, there may be a permanent, prominent bump at the dorsum of the finger where a lump of bone has formed at the fracture site.

JAMMED FINGER (MIDDLE PHALANX BASE AVULSION FRACTURE, VOLAR PLATE INJURY)

A common sports injury occurs when a ball hits the tip of the finger forcing it backwards further than it was designed to move. There is a wide ligament, called a volar plate, on the palm side of a finger at the PIP joint. Volar is another term for the palm side and is the opposite of dorsal. The term plate refers to a wide piece of tissue, in this case a ligament connecting 2 bones. When the finger is bent back and pressure applied to this ligament, it can only stretch so far. If the ligament does not tear, it can cause a fracture at the base of the middle phalanx. This is best seen on the lateral view of a finger radiograph. It looks like a little piece of bone has been chipped off the rest of the phalanx and is called an avulsion fracture (**Fig. 8**A). If the middle phalanx with avulsion fracture at the base is also subluxed (partially dislocated), this will require a surgical repair. Verify that the dorsal edges of the middle and proximal phalanges line up (**Fig. 8**B).

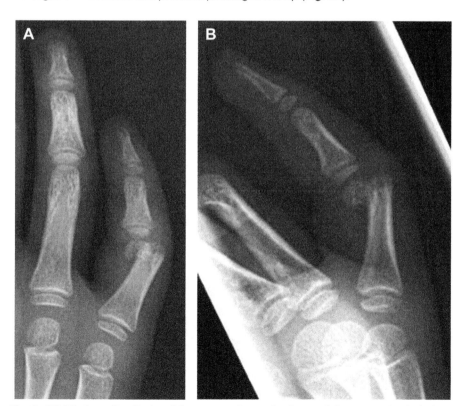

Fig. 9. (*A*) PA view of a displaced fracture at the neck of a small finger proximal phalanx. This is an unstable fracture, and a surgical pinning is required for this to heal properly. (*B*) Lateral radiographic view of a displaced small finger proximal phalanx neck fracture.

The most common mistake made when treating a jammed finger with a volar plate injury is to place it in a cast for 4 weeks. This causes the finger to become stiff because of the scar tissue that forms at the PIP joint. The best treatment for this injury is to splint the affected finger with an aluminum splint that has a curve of about 30°, which matches the normal bend of a finger at rest. The objective is to prevent this finger from being bent backwards during the healing process. This aluminum splint is worn for 1 week. For the following 3 weeks, the affected finger is buddy taped to a finger next to it. This provides a natural splint with the support of a noninjured finger. It also encourages the injured finger to move to reduce stiffness and improve range of motion. After 3 weeks of buddy taping, usually the injured finger has enough stability and strength so the patient is able to be released to full activity with no restrictions. This injury is managed alternatively with just buddy taping for 4 weeks without using the aluminum splint for the first week. During the 4-week healing process, contact sports should be avoided to decrease the risk of reinjuring the finger.

PROXIMAL PHALANX FRACTURE

The finger bone in closest proximity to the body is called the proximal phalanx. Fractures at the neck of a proximal phalanx (narrow end of the bone shaft closest to the fingernail) tend to be unstable and should be evaluated within the first week of the injury (**Fig. 9**). Surgery is required if the finger is malrotated or the distal bone fragment has become displaced (**Fig. 10**).[2]

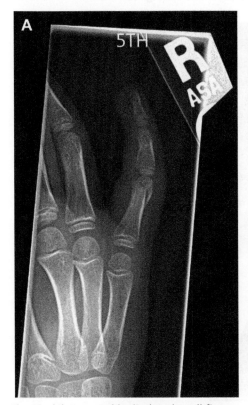
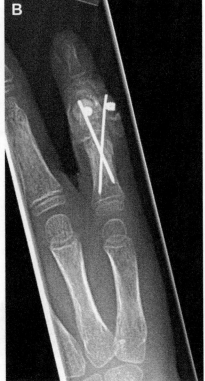

Fig. 10. (A) An unstable displaced small finger proximal phalanx neck fracture before surgical pinning. (B) A small finger proximal phalanx neck fracture after pinning.

Fractures at the base (bone end closest to the palm) of the proximal phalanx shaft tend to be more stable and heal well with protection in an ulnar gutter or cobra cast for 4 weeks. An ulnar gutter cast captures either the small and ring or small, ring, and middle fingers, while a cobra cast captures all 4 fingers. The choice between these casts depends on which finger is fractured. The cobra cast is appropriate to protect any of the smaller fingers for children younger than 6 years. Treatment for an extraoctave pinky fracture (**Fig. 11**) includes reducing the fracture, buddy taping the small and ring fingers, obtaining radiographs to confirm proper alignment, and then referring the child to a hand specialist within 48 hours.

Fractures at the base of the thumb proximal phalanx are a special case. If the thumb proximal phalanx bone fragment is below the joint line, then it should be evaluated by a surgeon. If the bone fragment is above the joint line, then it can be placed in a thumb spica cast for 4 weeks. If there is malrotation in any finger (assessed by comparing the way the finger nail is facing compared with the other fingers or the other thumb) or angulation (all fingers should point toward the scaphoid when flexed), this injury should also be evaluated by a surgeon. Surgical repairs should be done within the first 2 weeks after finger fractures.

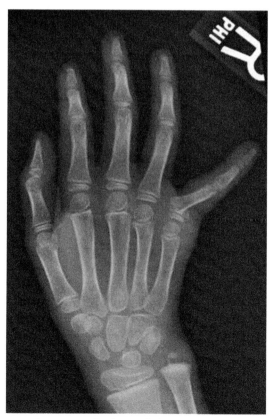

Fig. 11. An extraoctave fracture at the base of the small finger proximal phalanx comes from piano terminology meaning the new angle enables one to reach 8 more piano notes. This should be seen by a hand specialist within 48 hours.

FINGER DISLOCATIONS

The small finger is especially prone to dislocations from impacting balls or getting caught in sports clothing (**Fig. 12**). Early reduction is beneficial to the soft tissue at the joint including ligaments, nerves, blood vessels, and cartilage. After reducing the dislocation, if sensation is lost or blood is not reaching the fingertip, this should be urgently evaluated at the emergency department. Treatment for a reduced finger dislocation includes buddy taping the finger and protecting it in a splint for 3 weeks. The splint should extend past the joints on both sides of the dislocated joint to be effective.

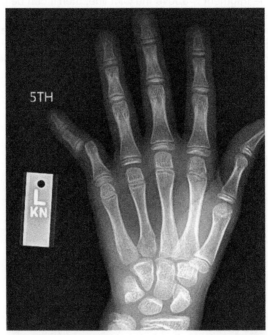

Fig. 12. This is a dislocation at the PIP joint of the left pinky from catching it on a football jersey.

TRIGGER THUMB

Some young children develop a thumb that snaps or triggers when flexed and extended, which may progress to getting caught in a flexed position. Although the exact cause of a trigger thumb is unclear, some speculate that a fall may have caused the initial insult to the flexor tendon, causing a fibrous nodule, or bump, to form. Although every child falls, fortunately not every child develops a trigger thumb.

There is a tunnel of tissue at the base of the thumb through which the flexor tendon slides when bending the thumb. This tunnel is called the A1 pulley. When a small bump forms in the flexor tendon, it catches on this tunnel, causing a snapping or triggering motion in the thumb. If this bump gets bigger, it can get caught on one side of the tunnel, typically causing the thumb to be held in a flexed, or bent, position at the interphalangeal (IP) joint (**Fig. 13**).

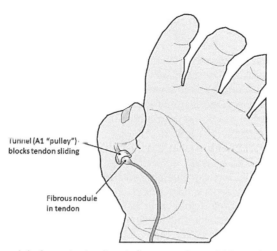

Fig. 13. A fibrous nodule forms in the thumb flexor tendon, which catches on the A1 pulley.

A trigger thumb is a different process from adult trigger fingers. In children, a fibrous nodule forms in the flexor tendon that gets caught on the A1 pulley at the base of the finger. In adults, there is an inflammatory process with swelling that affects the flexor tendon causing it to catch on the A1 pulley. As a result, treatment for adults and children with trigger fingers is different. For example, steroid injections are never used in children's hands because of the risk of a tendon rupture but may help reduce swelling in adults.

When a thumb is noticed to be snapping or permanently flexed at the IP joint (**Fig. 14**A), one can place a finger at the base of the thumb on the palm side and feel for a lump under the skin. Pressure on this bump should not be painful. Flexing and extending the tip of the thumb should cause this lump to move back and forth under the examiner's finger. If a mobile lump is discovered, there is no need for radiograph or ultrasound imaging. This condition is often present for a while before a parent notices it, because it does not hurt the child and does not limit daily activities.

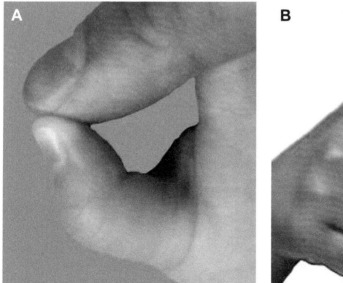
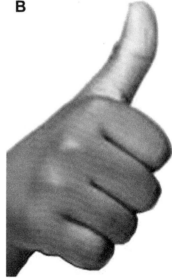

Fig. 14. (*A*) Pressure at the tip of a blocked trigger thumb does not cause it to extend fully without pain. (*B*) The normal range of motion of the thumb when the flexor tendon can slide freely.

When previous family photos of the child are examined, the bent thumb is often found to be present for weeks or months before it was first noticed.

Although numerous approaches have been tried to fix a trigger thumb including bracing, acupuncture, and massage, if the triggering has not resolved by the age of 4 years, then a surgical solution is warranted. This is the most common surgical procedure performed by a hand surgeon.

A child with a trigger thumb should just be monitored until the age range of 2 to 4. A surgical procedure is not typically done until the child turns 2 when risks associated with general anesthesia are significantly reduced. Reduced thumb range of motion because of a thumb caught in a flexed position can result in thumb IP joint deformity if left untreated. If the triggering goes away before the child turns 4, then nothing needs to be done (**Fig. 14**B). For Seattle Children's Hospital patients with trigger thumb, up to 14% percent of the time both thumbs get caught in a flexed position. Waiting until the child is between the ages of 2 and 4 years also gives time to see if both thumbs are going to trigger. And if so, both can be released during the same surgical procedure. The procedure involves enlarging the tunnel space under the A1 pulley rather than trying to remove the nodule, which could result in a tendon rupture.

CLINODACTYLY

Some children may be born with fingers, typically both pinkies, that curve toward the thumb. Initially this curve may be subtle and not noticed by the parents. It may first come to the parent's attention after a fall with pain in the pinky. Radiographic imaging of these fingers can be confused with a crush injury to the middle phalanx (**Fig. 15**A).

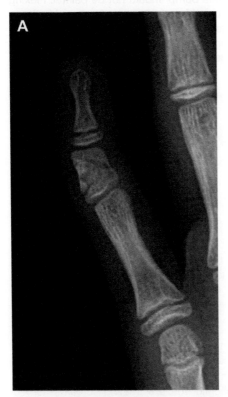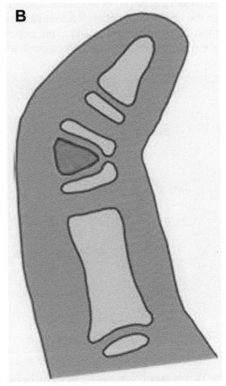

Fig. 15. (A) With clinodactyly, the middle phalanx has an odd shape that causes the pinky to curve. (B) The delta phalanx (*blue*) is a bracketed epiphysis with 2 growth plates.

However, clinodactyly is a congenital deformity that occurs when the middle phalanx of the small finger has 2 growth plates instead of 1, which creates a trapezoidal or triangular-shaped bone instead of a rectangle (**Fig. 15**B). This is a variant of normal. A mild deflection of the pinky fingertip toward the thumb should cause no pain or disability. If this curve becomes more severe, it is best to have the child evaluated by a surgeon. Any correction of this curve should be delayed until late childhood to reduce the risk of the deformity developing again.

GANGLION CYST

Bumps sometimes form at the wrist that can be caused by repetitive activities, injuries to the wrist joint capsule or tendon sheath, or for no clear reason. These bumps can be a result of a fluid-filled cyst, a soft tissue tumor, or an abnormal growth of blood vessels (called a vascular malformation). A cyst forms when there is a weak area in the joint capsule tissue. The fluid in the wrist joint is under a lot of pressure and can push up this weak tissue to create a fluid-filled balloon, or cyst. Cysts can also form from a weak spot in a tendon sheath. The fluid that lubricates the tendon is also under pressure and can create a balloon anywhere along the tube that surrounds the tendon. These can be found from the wrist to the fingers. Ganglion cysts at the wrist tend to be mobile, sliding around under the skin since they are not attached to the skin.

A quick and inexpensive way to distinguish a cyst from other causes of the bump can be done using the otoscope light usually found on the wall of a clinic examination room. Place the light at 1 side of the bump and see if a shadow forms preventing the

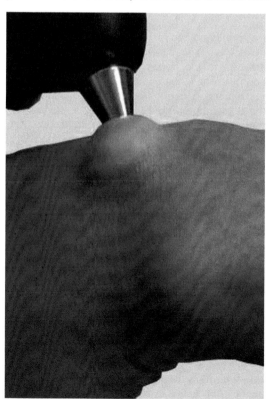

Fig. 16. If light fills the entire bump with transillumination, this indicates a fluid-filled ganglion cyst. Firmer tissue would create a shadow.

light from permeating the entire area of tissue. This technique is called transillumination (**Fig. 16**). If there is no shadow, this is likely a ganglion cyst. For a definitive diagnosis, an ultrasound can be ordered.

The wrist bump may be present for a long period of time before it is brought in to be evaluated. If the bump is not causing any aggravating symptoms, the best course of action is to monitor the bump for at least the next 3 months. Fifty percent of the time these bumps will go away on their own.

If the bump grows big enough that it restricts the wrist's range of motion, limits activities of daily living, or is causing pain because of its position near a nerve, then the bump should be evaluated by a hand surgeon. Removing these bumps surgically is not done lightly. Up to 21% of the time these bumps can return after the surgical excision procedure.[3] If the surgery is unsuccessful, the child has gone from having a bump on the wrist to having a scar and a bump.

If parents have been doing some research on the Internet or are familiar with how ganglion cysts are treated in adults, you might hear questions about "why are you not proposing to remove the fluid from the cyst using a needle to aspirate the bump" or "why not inject a steroid into the area to reduce inflammation?" In children, aspirating a cyst or doing a steroid injection is scary because of needle phobia and often result in the bump returning. In addition, children's tendons are extremely sensitive to steroids and can break down, causing tendon rupture with just 1 injection. This could create devastating complications requiring multiple surgical procedures that generate scar tissue and cause stiffness.

SCAPHOID FRACTURE

Falls onto an outstretched hand can result in fractures to the bones in the hand, wrist, and forearm. Whenever there is wrist pain following a traumatic injury, always check to see if there is a fracture to the bones in the wrist (the carpal bones). The most commonly broken carpal bone is the scaphoid.[4]

During the physical examination, put pressure on the anatomic snuffbox at the base of the thumb on the dorsal side (**Fig. 17**A). If there is point tenderness, make sure radiographic imaging of the wrist includes the scaphoid view. If a scaphoid fracture is missed, this can result in chronic wrist pain. It is common for scaphoid fractures to not show up if the radiograph is done right after the injury. Repeat a child's radiographs in 1 week or a teenager in 2 weeks if there is a suspected scaphoid fracture. By that time the resorption process should have removed enough damaged bone for the fracture to become visible (**Fig. 17**B).

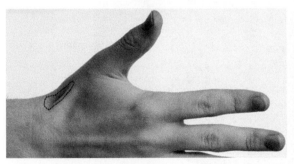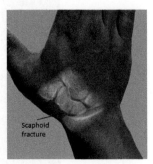

Fig. 17. (*A*) The anatomic snuffbox is formed between the extensor pollicis longus and brevis tendons of the thumb. (*B*) Pressure at this indentation of the anatomic snuffbox will be tender if the scaphoid is broken.

A nondisplaced scaphoid fracture can be placed in a thumb spica short arm cast for 6 weeks. If repeated radiographs in 6 weeks show a normal healing process, then the patient can transition to a thumb spica brace for another 2 weeks. The brace is worn full-time and only removed for showering and eating. Scaphoid fractures that are displaced or are not healing well should be evaluated by an orthopedic hand surgeon.

DISTAL RADIUS AND ULNA FRACTURES

Falls onto outstretched arms often cause broken bones in the forearm. If the radius, on the thumb side of the forearm, is broken near the wrist but not displaced or angulated, it can be treated well in a short-arm cast for 4 weeks. Radiographic imaging, using posterior-anterior (PA) and lateral views, should be repeated about 1 week after the initial injury if the fracture is angulated or if a displaced fracture has been reduced. If there is bone movement at 1 week, then imaging should be done again at 2 weeks. If the change in displacement or angulation is significant, this may require a reduction under sedation in the emergency department. At 1 week, a cast can be applied with molds that prevent more bone movement. These molds need to apply pressure to the distal end of the bone and must take into account whether the distal fragment is going to move volarly, dorsally, radially, or ulnarly. A flexion mold curving toward the palm, for example, can prevent the distal fragment from shifting dorsally. The curve of the mold should start at the level of the fracture to be effective. Two weeks after the initial injury, fractures tend to become stable. A long-arm cast should be considered if the initial fracture required a reduction, if both bones in the forearm are broken, or if the child is less than 2 years of age (in very young children there is an increased risk of the short arm cast sliding off the arm because of the shape of the anatomy with a carrot-shaped forearm and negligible wrist).

If radiographic imaging shows that there is normal bone healing with callus formation and periosteal reaction around 4 weeks after the initial injury, children can transition to a wrist brace that is worn for another 2 weeks. If there is angulation at the fracture site, the brace can be worn longer until remodeling decreases the angulation. The brace is worn full-time and only removed for bathing and eating. The main objective of the brace is to continue to protect the healing broken bone and prevent muscle strains. It is removed for short periods of time so the wrist range of motion can improve.

During the entire 6 to 7 weeks in the cast and brace the child should refrain from contact sports. On physical activity notes, the author typically writes "No balls (eg, dodgeball, football), no wheels (eg, bicycles, scooters, skates), and keep both feet on the ground (ie, avoid monkey bars and trampolines)."

Distal radius fractures, near the wrist, will remodel 10% per year until the child reaches puberty. The acceptable amount of angulation at the fracture site varies depending on the age of the child. For children up to 5 years of age, the angulation does not need to be reduced if it is less than 20°. Children between 5 and 10 years old can tolerate angulation less than 15°. And children 10 to 15 years old do not need a reduction if the angle is less than 10°.[5]

The terminology used to describe a bone fracture angle can sometimes be confusing. One way to provide clarity is to use the term apex. When an angle is created at a bone fracture site, this forms the shape of an arrow. The apex is the point or tip of that arrow. If the arrow is pointing toward the palm, or volar, side of the wrist, then that would be described as an apex volar angulation (**Fig. 18**). Apex dorsal angulation describes the arrow pointing to the back of the wrist. If the arrow points toward the thumb side of the wrist, one would describe that as apex radial angulation. Apex ulnar angulation describes an arrow that points toward the pinky side of the wrist (**Fig. 19**).

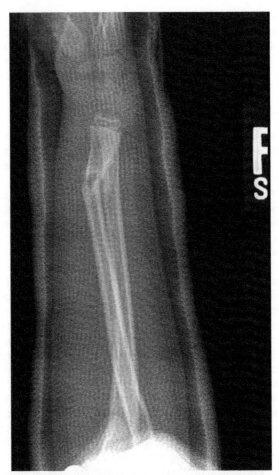

Fig. 18. The arrow tip at this fracture points to the left, which is the volar or palm side of the arm. This would be described as an apex volar angulation. The cast was applied without a curve toward the palm side (a flexion mold) and thus the distal bone fragment fell dorsally.

There is a special type of distal radius fracture pattern that occurs in young children called a buckle or torus fracture. These terms refer to a process where the edge of the bone, the cortical surface, is stretched on one side during a traumatic injury that causes a bump to form on that side (**Fig. 20**A). There should be no angulation seen on the lateral radiographic view of the wrist with a simple buckle fracture (**Fig. 20**B). If bumps form on both sides of the bone (**Fig. 21**), that is treated differently than a simple buckle fracture. It is important to recognize that a radiologist's report may identify a buckle fracture that does not meet this criteria of a simple buckle fracture. Instead of using a cast, a simple buckle fracture can be placed in a wrist brace with Velcro straps for 4 weeks. The brace should be kept dry and only removed for bathing during this 4-week period. At the end of 4 weeks, the child does not need to return to the clinic, as there is no cast to be removed. No additional radiographic imaging is needed unless a new traumatic event has caused a new injury.[6]

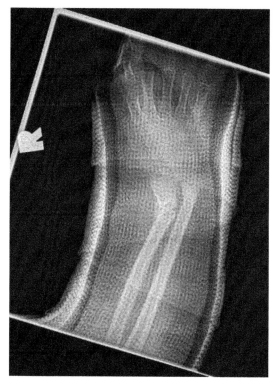

Fig. 19. This distal radius fracture points toward the ulna and is said to have apex ulnar angulation. This cast should have had an ulnar deviation mold to try and prevent the distal radius from tipping to the radial side.

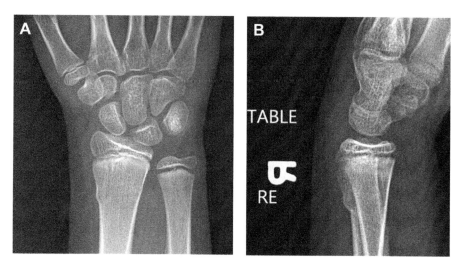

Fig. 20. (*A*) A simple buckle fracture only has 1 bump (buckle) on the side of the radius. This is the PA radiographic view. (*B*) On the lateral radiographic view, a simple buckle fracture has no angulation (the distal fragment does not tip to one side). This type of fracture can be treated in a brace, instead of a cast, for 4 weeks with no need to return to the clinic.

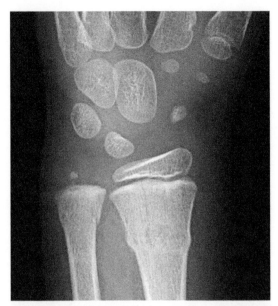

Fig. 21. When bumps occur on both sides of a bone (seen in this radius) or there is disruption of the cortical surface (seen on the radial side of the distal ulna), these fractures should be managed in a cast.

There is an increased risk of a growth plate closing early causing deformity with certain types of fractures (**Fig. 22**). Patients with displaced fractures at the growth plate or Salter-Harris three (fracture from the growth plate to the joint surface), four (fracture through the growth plate to the joint surface), and five (crush injury to the growth plate) fractures should return at 6 months after the initial injury for a growth plate, or physis, check. If the child is going through a growth spurt, it would be prudent to have him or her return at 3 months after the injury. If the growth plate is not clearly and completely open, this child should be referred to an orthopedic surgeon.

Injuries to the ligament at the distal radius and ulna joint (DRUJ) are rare in children. If there is instability at this joint when the forearm is in pronation (palm facing down) yet this joint becomes stable in supination, this child should be referred to a hand surgeon for evaluation.

RADIUS AND ULNA SHAFT FRACTURES

Most bone growth in the forearm occurs near the growth plates at the wrist. As a result, fractures that occur in the shaft (diaphysis) of the radius and ulna take longer to heal than when the bone is broken close to the wrist (**Fig. 23**A). PA and lateral radiographs should be obtained at 1 and 2 weeks after the initial injury to ensure that proper anatomic alignment is being maintained. At the 1-week visit, a fracture that has been reduced can have the splint overwrapped with fiberglass material to provide more stability if alignment is being maintained. At 2 weeks, a new long-arm cast can be applied if the splint is loose on the arm. The cast should be applied for at least the first 6 weeks. A forearm brace can replace the cast if there is evidence of good healing with

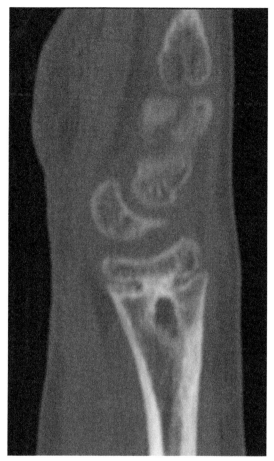

Fig. 22. A computed tomography scan captured early closure of a growth plate with a physeal bar in the middle connecting the epiphysis to the metaphysis. This needs to be evaluated by a surgeon for management.

callus formation and periosteal reaction. The brace is worn for at least 2 weeks and potentially longer if remodeling is required to achieve anatomic alignment (**Fig. 23**B).

Based on the most recent research, there is up to a 5% chance (1 out of every 20 cases) of breaking forearm bones a second time, in the same place. There is a higher risk to break these bones again if the first fracture is in the middle of the forearm bones (see **Fig. 23**A). Most repeat fractures tend to happen within 6 months after the first injury.[7,8]

Wearing a cast for at least 6 weeks followed by a brace for another 2 to 4 weeks reduces the risk of breaking the same arm bones again. The metal plates in the brace continue to protect the injured area and start improving wrist movement when the brace is removed for bathing and at meal times. While the child wears a brace, he or she should not participate in contact sports (eg, soccer, football, or dodge ball). Gymnastics, contact sports, and full weight-bearing on the affected arm (eg, push-ups) should be avoided for 6 months following a forearm bone shaft fracture with angulation.

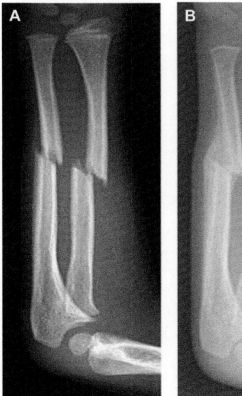
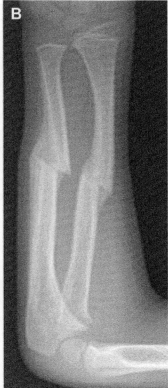

Fig. 23. (*A*) Radiographs just after a traumatic injury with fractures at the middle of the shaft of the radius and ulna in the forearm. (*B*) Radiographs of both bone, midshaft forearm fractures at around 6 weeks showing callus filling in the gaps as part of the remodeling process.

MONTEGGIA AND GALIAZZI FRACTURE DISLOCATIONS

Whenever a fracture occurs in the shaft of a forearm bone, the alignment at the nearest joint should be scrutinized for a dislocation. A fracture of the shaft of the ulna near the elbow with a radial head dislocation is called a Monteggia fracture dislocation (**Fig. 24**). A Galiazzi fracture dislocation combines a broken radius bone near the wrist with a dislocation of the ulna at the DRUJ (**Fig. 25**). These fracture dislocations need to be treated at the emergency department, because reducing the dislocation is painful when combined with a bone fracture and requires sedation.

SUMMARY

Many traumatic injuries of the hand and forearm can be treated in primary care. Injury treatment protocols discussed here should help to avoid overtreating volar plate injuries and decrease the risk of stiffness. Recognizing injuries at high risk for infection, like a Seymour fracture; high risk for chronic pain, as seen with scaphoid fractures and finger dislocations; or at high risk for healing with a deformity, such as unstable distal radius fractures and Galiazzi and Monteggia fracture dislocations should avoid long-term complications by referring them for specialist evaluation. Matching the severity of

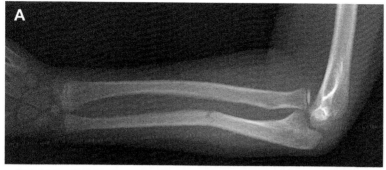

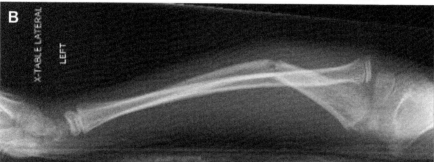

Fig. 24. (*A*) This is a Monteggia ulna fracture dislocation. The radial head at the elbow is dislocated. It should be aligned with the capitellum, the round knob at the base of the humerus bone. Note, the radius is dislocated anteriorly. (*B*) This is a Monteggia ulna fracture dislocation. In this example, the radial head at the elbow is dislocated posteriorly.

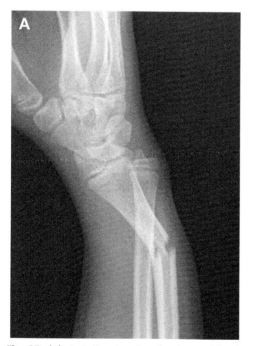 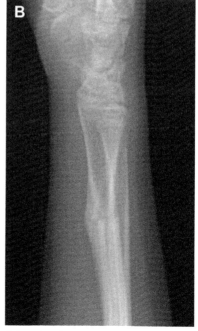

Fig. 25. (*A*) A Galiazzi radius fracture with ulna dislocation has the ulna not lining up behind the radius in the lateral radiographic view, because it is dislocated posteriorly at the DRUJ. (*B*) After reduction of a Galiazzi radius fracture with ulna dislocation, this looks like a normal healing radius fracture.

the traumatic arm injury to the appropriate treatment can facilitate children getting back to their primary job of playing and learning.

DISCLOSURE

This author has nothing to disclose.

REFERENCES

1. Arora R, Fichadia U, Hartwig E, et al. Pediatric upper-extremity fractures. Pediatr Ann 2014;43(5):196–204.
2. Cornwall R, Ricchetti ET. Pediatric phalanx fractures: unique challenges and pitfalls. Clin Orthop Relat Res 2006;445:146–56.
3. Head L, Gencarelli JR, Allen M, et al. Wrist ganglion treatment: systematic review and meta-analysis. J Hand Surg Am 2015;40(3):546–53.
4. Li H, Guo W, Guo S, et al. Surgical versus nonsurgical treatment for scaphoid waist fracture with slight or no displacement: A meta-analysis and systematic review. Medicine (Baltimore) 2018;97(48):e13266.
5. Thompson JC. Netter's concise orthopaedic anatomy. Incomplete fracture treatment. 2nd edition. Saunders Elsevier; 2010.
6. Kuba MHM, Izuka BH. One brace: one visit: treatment of pediatric distal radius buckle fractures with a removable wrist brace and no follow-up visit. J Pediatr Orthop 2018;38:e338–42.
7. Bould M, Bannister GC. Refractures of the radius and ulna in children. Injury 1999; 30:583–6.
8. Tisosky AJ, Werger MM, McPartland TG, et al. The factors influencing the refracture of pediatric forearms. J Pediatr Orthop 2015;35:677–81.

Toe Walking

Review of the Differential Diagnosis and Treatment Options to Ensure Optimal Gross Motor Development

John Forrest Bennett, MN, ARNP[a], Jaclyn Omura, MD[b],*

KEYWORDS

- Toe walking • Gross motor development • Orthotics • Therapies

KEY POINTS

- Toe walking is a common variation in gait.
- Clinicians must approach this gait abnormality with caution.
- An intentional history and physical examination can narrow a differential diagnosis and guide diagnostics as well as treatment.

INTRODUCTION

Toe walking is a common variation in gait in the developing child, indicates a neurologic injury to the central nervous system, or can even be a sign of progressive muscle wasting disease. The incidence of toe walking is between 2% and 5.5%.[1,2] The differential for toe walking is broad; therefore, a clinician must approach this gait abnormality with caution. A thorough and intentional history and physical examination can efficiently narrow a differential diagnosis, rule out diagnoses, and guide both diagnostics as well as treatment plans. The goal of this article is to help the general practitioner develop differential diagnosis for toe walking, identify appropriate initial diagnostics, recognize treatment algorithms, and understand how age and range of motion influences evaluation.

---

[a] Physical Medicine Rehabilitation, Mary Bridge Children's Hospital, PO Box 5299, MS: 311-1-PMR, 311 South L Street, Tacoma, WA 98415-0299, USA; [b] Rehabilitation Medicine, Seattle Children's Hospital, University of Washington School of Medicine, 4800 Sand Point Way Northeast, Seattle, WA 98105, USA
* Corresponding author.
E-mail address: Jaclyn.Omura@seattlechildrens.org

Physician Assist Clin 5 (2020) 477–485
https://doi.org/10.1016/j.cpha.2020.06.002
2405-7991/20/© 2020 Elsevier Inc. All rights reserved.
physicianassistant.theclinics.com

TYPICAL GAIT DEVELOPMENT

When discussing abnormal gait one must understand normal gait development. The typical age of walking is variable and influenced by several factors, although generally ranges between 10 and 18 months. Toddler gait patterns are immature and develop into a more mature gait cycle by the time they are 5 to 7 years old.[3] A typical toddler gait pattern consists of short step length, high cadence, wide base of support, pelvic tilt, with knees flexed, foot flat initial contact, and limited dorsiflexion during swing phase of the gait cycle. A reciprocal arm swing is not expected and most of their gait cycle is in double stance. Form follows function, as this toddler gait pattern reflects an underdeveloped neurologic system, poor motor control, and a disproportionately large head, when compared with the torso and extremities.

By 2 years of age, the toddler's gait pattern begins to change, reflecting critical development in motor control and body mechanics. Pelvic tilt decreases, the base of support narrows, time spent in single stance increases, and the toddler begins to achieve full knee extension in terminal stance, with emergence of both heel strike as well as reciprocal arm swing.[3] During this developmental window, toe walking is a typical developmental variant.

By 7 years of age, the school-age child has developed a mature gait pattern.[3] This consists of a shoulder width base of support, heel strike initial contact, toe off with full knee extension at terminal stance, full knee extension at terminal swing, and reciprocal arm swing. There does remain some age-specific variance of gait including a higher cadence, lower speed, slightly increased pelvic rotation, and abduction.

ATYPICAL GAIT: TOE WALKING

Toe walking can present from toddler age up to early adolescence. It can be a variant of normal gait but also can be a sign of underlying neurologic or muscle disorder, prompting referral to pediatric neurology, rehabilitation medicine, or orthopedics.

Patients who toe walk do not have consistent heel strike at initial contact, but their gait patterns can vary significantly. They commonly are described as having a toe–toe gait pattern, but the degree of their toe walking can range from having foot flat initial contact with early heel rise to walking on the foremost part of their foot. The time spent toe walking can also vary considerably, where some children are able to heel strike part of the time and other children walk with a toe-toe pattern 100% of the time.

Idiopathic toe walking is a diagnosis of exclusion. The differential diagnosis of toe walking must take into consideration several possible causes. There are 4 major categories of diagnoses to consider when evaluating these patients: upper motor neuron (UMN) pathology, neuromuscular pathology, developmental disorders, and orthopedic pathology. The history and physical examination are the most important part of evaluation, as they guide diagnostic workup and treatment decisions. A list of the most common diagnoses can be found in **Table 1**.

The history should be thorough and includes the following: toe walking history, developmental history, current function (gross motor, fine motor, language, and social skills), bowel/bladder function, birth history, past medical history, and family history. Concerning findings suggest underlying pathology will be discussed by category of diagnosis discussed in the next section. Despite potential cause, a diligent history about their toe walking must be obtained. This should include the following questions:

- When did the toe walking start?
- What percent of the time do they spend on their toes?

Table 1
Diagnosis categories to consider when evaluating a patient for toe walking

Upper motor neuron
  Cerebral palsy
  Traumatic brain injury
  Spinal cord injury
  Intracranial mass
  Tethered cord[a]
  Spina bifida[a]
	Lower motor neuron
	  Peripheral neuropathy
	  Myopathic process (ie, DMD, SMA, etc.)
	  Spinal muscular atrophy

Developmental disorder
  Autism spectrum disorder
  Sensory processing disorder
	Orthopedic pathology
	  Club foot
	  Developmental dysplasia of the hip
	  Hip or knee contracture

[a] Can present with upper motor or lower motor neuron findings.

- Is the patient able to get their heels on the ground at all while walking or while standing still?
- Has the patient undergone any prior workup or intervention (ie stretching, physical therapy, bracing)
- Any family history of toe walking?

The examination for toe walking should also always include a thorough neuro and lower extremity musculoskeletal (MSK) examination, including ankle dorsiflexion range of motion (normal is 15–20°) with knee flexed and knee extended (Silfverskiold test). This test evaluates which muscles in the calf may be tight and can help to guide treatment decisions.[4] A gait evaluation is also important, particularly paying attention to their initial contact, stride length, base of support, pelvic position, and arm swing. A quick way to assess ankle range of motion is to have the child perform a deep squat. The ability to perform a deep squat is correlated with ankle range of motion, where reduced ankle dorsiflexion limits depth of the squat.[5] Further evaluation of motor skills and coordination depends on age and can be accomplished with observation of single leg stance, single leg squat, and jumping.

The remainder of discussion related to evaluation and diagnostics is broken down by category.

UPPER MOTOR NEURON CAUSE: EVALUATION AND DIAGNOSTICS

The most common UMN cause associated with toe walking is cerebral palsy (CP). Less common causes include stroke, traumatic brain injury, tethered spinal cord, and spina bifida (although tethered cord and spina bifida can present with a lower motor neuron picture).

- History: pertinent findings and red flags
  - Toe walking history: toe walking on predominately one side is concerning for hemiplegic CP
  - Developmental history: delayed motor milestone achievement and early hand dominance is concerning for hemiplegic CP, early head control concerning for CP (due to hypertonicity in the neck extensors)
  - Birth history: the number one risk factor for CP is prematurity; other risk factors include prenatal exposures (medications, illegal substances), pre/perinatal infection, and low apgar scores[6]

- o History of trauma
- o Rapidly progressing scoliosis with changes in foot structure or new bowel/bladder issues should raise concern for tethered cord
- o Family history: spina bifida (risk to fetus increases with positive family history)
- Physical examination: pertinent findings and red flags
  - o HEENT: microcephaly or macrocephaly concerning for CP or acquired brain injury.
  - o Skin: sacral dimple or tuft of hair over the lumbar spine concerning for spina bifida.
  - o MSK: positive galeazzi indicates hip dysplasia, which can be seen in CP or spina bifida, typically due to an imbalance of musculature around the hip. Limb length discrepancy can be seen in hemiplegic CP. Dorsiflexion range of motion may be limited due to contracture in any UMN pathology.
  - o Neuroexamination: hyperreflexia, clonus, positive babinski, and spasticity can be seen in any UMN injury. Dystonia (abnormal posturing in the extremities, trunk, neck or face) is seen in CP or other acquired brain injury. Decreased sensation can be seen in CP or acquired brain injury.
  - o Spine: rapidly progressing scoliosis concerning for tethered cord.
  - o Gait: high toe–toe pattern with scissoring and/or flexed knee throughout gait cycle suggests increased muscle tone.
- Diagnostic workup: considerations
  - o Brain MRI to rule out CP or acquired brain injury
  - o Spine MRI (depending on examination can be total spine or more specific) to rule out spina bifida, tethered cord, or spinal cord injury
  - o Referral to a neurologist or rehabilitation medicine specialist is warranted if you have concerns about an UMN cause in patients with persistent toe walking

NEUROMUSCULAR: EVALUATION AND DIAGNOSTICS

A variety of neuromuscular diagnoses present with toe walking that typically starts in early childhood. The most common of these diagnoses is duchenne muscular dystrophy (DMD), but differential includes spinal muscular atrophy type III and limb girdle muscular dystrophy. Peripheral neuropathies such as Charcot-Marie-Tooth (CMT) can also present with toe walking in childhood or early adolescence.

- History: pertinent findings and red flags
  - o Toe walking history: toe walking that was not present when patient first started walking or is getting more significant. History of frequent falls concerning for muscle weakness.
  - o Developmental history: delayed motor milestone achievement and delayed language skills or social/emotional skills can be seen in boys with DMD. Difficulty getting up off the floor is also concerning for proximal weakness.
  - o Birth history: some patients with neuromuscular disorders require neonatal intensive care unit stay for feeding difficulty or respiratory support.
  - o History of decreased sensation starting in the feet concerning for peripheral neuropathy.
  - o Family history: muscular dystrophy (especially when evaluating a boy with toe walking). CMT is hereditary, and often there is a positive family history of pes cavus or abnormal gait.
- Physical examination: pertinent findings and red flags
  - o MSK: calf pseudohypertrophy seen in DMD. Muscle wasting or loss of foot intrinsic musculature in peripheral neuropathy.

- o Neuroexamination: bulbar weakness, absent reflexes, proximal weakness concerning for muscular dystrophy. Distal weakness and decreased sensation are concerning for peripheral neuropathy. Tongue fasciculations and tremor, along with muscle weakness, are concerning for spinal muscular atrophy.
- o Gait: a wide-based gait, positive Trendelenburg, and increased lumbar lordosis suggest proximal weakness. Foot drop or foot slap suggests distal weakness.
- o Positive gower's sign (rolling to prone before standing up from floor) concerning for proximal muscle weakness.[7]
- Diagnostic workup: considerations
  - o Creatine kinase (CK) level
  - o Referral for electromyography if concerned about peripheral neuropathy
  - o If high suspicion for neuromuscular disorder based on history, examination, or CK level, refer to neurology urgently

DEVELOPMENTAL DISORDERS: EVALUATION AND DIAGNOSTICS

Toe walking has been described as a common co-occurring condition in individuals with autism spectrum disorder and other developmental disorders. The American Academy of Pediatrics discourages providers using sensory processing disorder as a working diagnosis.[8] They encourage further workup of children identified to have challenges with sensory processing, including autism spectrum disorder, attention deficit disorder, and other developmental disorders. They also encourage close monitoring of sensory integration therapies for effective behavior or functional modulation.[8]

One study followed-up 954 patients in a developmental medicine clinic and found rates of persistent toe walking (defined as >3 months after independent ambulation) as high as 20.1% in patients with autism spectrum disorder.[9] Ankle dorsiflexion range of motion was limited in only 12.1% of patients.[9] This study did find lower rates of persistent toe walking among children with a diagnosis of Asperger syndrome, which is different from autism spectrum disorders, as children do not have language delay at 2 to 3 years of age. This study, and others, speculate that persistent toe walking reflects more severe language impairment.[9,10]

- History: pertinent findings and red flags
  - o Toe walking history: toe walking gets worse on cold surfaces, such as tile flooring, or uneven surfaces, such as grass or sand.
  - o Developmental history: children with developmental disorders can present with a wide variety of delay ranging from global delay to solely delays in social/emotional skills.
  - o Birth history: advanced parental age and gestational diabetes are identified risk factors for autism spectrum disorder.[11]
- Physical examination: pertinent findings and red flags
  - o MSK: normal, may have ankle dorsiflexion contractures
  - o Neuroexamination: normal
  - o Psych: children with autism spectrum disorder may avoid eye contact or exhibit repetitive behaviors
  - o Gait: variable, often these children are very high up on their toes with a short step length.
- Diagnostic workup: considerations
  - o Referral to neurodevelopmental pediatrician if high suspicion for developmental disorder

   ○ Referral to occupational therapy for further evaluation of developmental disorder

ORTHOPEDIC PATHOLOGY: EVALUATION AND DIAGNOSTICS

Orthopedic deformities are less likely to present with toe walking alone. The main diagnoses to consider are clubfoot, developmental hip dysplasia, and knee or hip flexion contractures. Developmental hip dysplasia is typically diagnosed in the neonate, although occasionally can be missed and can lead to toe walking or in-toeing in a child or adolescent.[12] The history is typically benign, with most pertinent findings on MSK examination of the lower extremity and foot. Again, a thorough evaluation of range of motion in the lower extremity joints is important, including Galeazzi, Barlow, and Ortolani hip maneuvers to rule out hip dysplasia.[12] If findings are abnormal, consider XR of the joint in question or referral to orthopedics.

CONTROVERSY OF TREATMENT

Treatment of idiopathic toe walking remains controversial. Eastwood and colleagues[13] noted that idiopathic toe walking is likely a persistent gait abnormality that improves with age that it is not dramatically altered by serial casting, although it may be responsive to surgery. This contradicts the Cincinnati Children's Hospital medical center's care guideline.[14] A more recent study noted that children with moderate to severe idiopathic toe walking demonstrated "significant improvements in ankle kinematics, ankle kinetics, and severity as adolescents and/or young adults" after being treated with casting and ankle-foot orthoses (AFOs).[15] The inclusion of gait laboratory data and the broader metrics suggests that prior studies may not have used metrics sensitive enough to capture the effect of active treatment with idiopathic toe walking.

Only 4 trials met the inclusion criteria of a Cochrane review in 2019, of which 3 trials did not provide results that could be included in the review.[16] They concluded that the evidence was too uncertain to determine if there were differences between serial casting with Botox injections, compared with serial casting alone. The review otherwise failed to comment on the broader treatment interventions of toe walking. Any attempt to standardize the treatment of idiopathic toe walking and to use objective metrics to track the efficacy of a treatment plan is crucial, given the relative lack of evidence.

TREATMENT OPTIONS

The Cincinnati care guideline targets patients with a confirmed diagnosis of idiopathic toe walking with no other contributing causes or red flags. At the time of publication, the Cincinnati care guideline was the most rigorous care guideline for this population and delineated treatment indications based upon age and available ankle range of motion.[14] Treatment options are listed in **Table 2**.

Table 2 Treatment options	
Nonsurgical	**Surgical**
• Physical therapy—stretching, strengthening, gait training, home exercise program • Daytime AFOs • Nighttime splint • Serial casting	• Tendo Achilles lengthening, gastrocnemius recession

When developing a plan of care, treatment should take into account the percentage of time a child walks on their toes, their available range of motion with leg extended, and the age of the child. Older children may not respond to stretching or serial casting as effectively as younger patients, although the research into most effective treatments is lacking. Thielemann and colleagues noted benefit from serial casting in a small cohort of patients aged between 5 and 15 years.[17] The Cincinnati Children's Hospital's care guideline makes no reference to age, with the treatment paradigm for idiopathic toe walking focused primarily on ankle dorsiflexion range of motion (**Fig. 1**).

For patients whom present with less than or equal to neutral (0) degrees of ankle dorsiflexion with passive range of motion, serial casting is recommended. Serial casting provides a persistent stretch to the gastrocnemius soleus complex performed by skilled physical therapist or orthopedic provider.[17] The goal of serial casting is to gain 5° of improved dorsiflexion per cast change, with the ultimate goal of having 5 to 10° of passive ankle dorsiflexion in standing. The number of casts required in this process varies, and contraindications for serial casting include the following:

- Impaired skin integrity
- Impaired circulation
- Lower extremity edema
- Recent fracture to extremity
- Decreased bone density
- Bony restriction at joint
- Hypermobile joints above or below
- Intolerance of procedure by patient

When considering serial casting, clinicians must proceed with caution in patients who have the following:

- Decreased sensation
- Decreased ability to communicate
- Poor cast compliance in the past
- Excessive sweating
- Patients at risk for fracture

The goal of serial casting is to increase ankle dorsiflexion range of motion, decrease toe walking frequency, and improve functional kinematic parameters. Serial casting

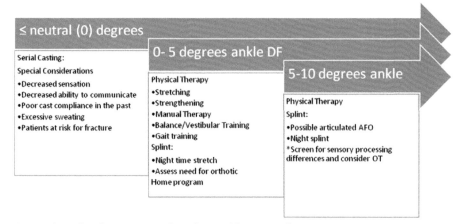

Fig. 1. Algorithm for treatment based on ankle range of motion.

can improve passive ankle dorsiflexion as well as functional kinematic parameters when followed by additional supportive treatment.[17–19]

For patients with 0 to 5° ankle dorsiflexion physical therapy is recommended. Frequency and duration of therapy depends on individual patient need. Skilled physical therapy will help establish a home program, teach stretches and range of motion exercises, and work on core strengthening, manual therapy, and gait training. Treatment may include the following:

- Kinesio taping
- Resting night splints
- Balance/vestibular training.

The treatment course for patients with 5 to 10° ankle dorsiflexion is similar to that for patients with 0 to 5° of dorsiflexion. Physical therapy is recommended. Frequency and duration of therapy depends on individual patient need. Treatment may include use of an articulated AFO and＼or resting night splint. The goals of therapy are to

- Increase ankle dorsiflexion
- Increase heel to pattern with and without the AFO
- Improve balance

Other treatments for toe walking include sensory processing interventions, sensory "diet," and prism glasses, which may warrant consideration. Some clinicians have noted the importance of screening for sensory processing challenges, although (as already stated) the AAP does not consider "sensory processing disorder" an appropriate diagnosis.[8]

SUMMARY

Toe walking is a common gait abnormality in pediatrics, which can be due to several causes. It is imperative that clinicians proceed cautiously when evaluating this gait abnormality and perform a consistent and intentional history and physical examination to screen for potentially progressive or more significant causes. When idiopathic toe walking is confirmed as the appropriate diagnosis, clinicians should provide anticipatory guidance regarding the limited evidence of treatment, while personalizing the plan of care.

DISCLOSURE

The authors have nothing to disclose.

REFERENCES

1. Engström P, Tedroff K. The prevalence and course of idiopathic toe-walking in 5-year-old children. Pediatrics 2012;130(2):279–84.
2. Engström P, Tedroff K. Idiopathic toe-walking: prevalence and natural history from birth to ten years of age. J Bone Joint Surg Am 2018;100(8):640–7.
3. Sutherland DH, Olshen R, Cooper L, et al. The development of mature gait. J Bone Joint Surg Am 1980;62(3):336–53.
4. Oetgen M, Peden S. Idiopathic toe walking. J Am Acad Orthop Surg 2012;20(5): 292–300.
5. Kasuyama T, Sakamoto M, Nakazawa R. Ankle joint dorsiflexion measurement using the deep squatting posture. J Phys Ther Sci 2009;21(2):195–9.

6. Graham HK, Thomason P, Novacheck TF, et al. Lovell & Winter's Pediatric Orthopaedics. Chapter 14: cerebral palsy. LWW 2016.
7. Wallace GB, Newton RW. Gowers' sign revisited. Arch Dis Child 1989;64(9): 1317–9.
8. Zimmer M, Desch L. Sensory integration therapies for children with developmental and behavioral disorders. The American Academy of Pediatrics 2012.
9. Barrow WJ, Jaworski M, Accardo PJ. Persistent toe walking in autism. J Child Neurol 2011;26(5):619–21.
10. Accardo P, Morrow J, Heaney MS, et al. Toe walking and language development. Clin Pediatr 1992;31(3):158–60.
11. Gardener H, Donna S, Buka S. Prenatal risk factors for autism: comprehensive meta-analysis. Br J Psychiatry 2009;195(1):7–14.
12. Aronsson D, Goldberg MJ, Kling TF Jr, et al. Developmental dysplasia of the hip. Pediatrics 1994;94(2):201–8.
13. Eastwood D, Menlaus M, Dickens R, et al. Idiopathic toe-walking: Does treatment alter the natural history? J Ped Orrthop B 2000;9:47–9.
14. Cincinnati Children's Hospital Medical Center. Evidence-based care guideline for management of idiopathic toe walking in children and young adults ages 2 through 21 years. Cincinnati (OH): Cincinnati Children's Hospital Medical Center; 2011.
15. Davies K, Black A, Hunt M, et al. Long-term gait outcomes following conservative management of idiopathic toe walking. Gait Posture 2018;62:214–9.
16. Caserta AJ, Pacey V, Fahey MC, et al. Interventions for Toe Walking. Cochrane Database for Systematic Van Juijk A et al. Treatment for idiopathic toe walking: A systematic review of the literature. J Rehabil Med 2014;46:945–57.
17. Thielemann F, Rockstroh G, Mehrholz J, et al. Serial ankle casts for patients with idiopathic toe walking: effects on functional gait parameters. J Child Orthop 2019; 13:147–54.
18. Van Juijk A, Kosters R, Vugts M, et al. Treatment for idiopathic toe walking: A systematic review of the literature. J Rehabil Med 2014;46:945–57.
19. Fox A, Deakin S, Pettigrew G, et al. Serial casting in the treatment of idiopathic toe-walkers and review of the literature. Acta Orthop Belg 2006;72(6):722–30.

Hip Dysplasia – Birth to 6 Months

Keith Lemay, PA-C*, Cheryl Parker, PA-C, Todd Blumberg, MD

KEYWORDS

- Hip • Dysplasia • Dislocation • Pavlik • Developmental dysplasia of the hip
- Ortolani • Barlow • Ultrasound

KEY POINTS

- Developmental hip dysplasia is the most common musculoskeletal conditions affecting newborns.
- Breech position during pregnancy and family history are significant risk factors.
- Treatment with a Pavlik harness at a young age significantly improves the patient's hip joint durability.

 Video content accompanies this article at http://www.physicianassistant.theclinics.com.

Developmental dysplasia of the hip (DDH) is the most common newborn orthopedic disorder. The incidence of dysplasia is 11.5 cases per 1000 births, and frank dislocation occurs at a rate of 1.5 cases per 1000 births.[1,2] In DDH, the body fails to properly form a ball and socket joint. It encompasses a spectrum of severity from mild ultrasonographic dysplasia to irreducible hip dislocation. Failure to recognize and treat DDH may result in a limb length discrepancy, knee deformity, and/or degenerative hip arthritis in early adulthood.[3,4]

The exact etiology of DDH is unknown. It is thought to be a multifactorial packaging disorder. In utero, the hip joint is formed when the pelvis and the femoral head are in contact with each other.[5,6] Both anatomic factors of the fetus and environmental factors of the uterus affect the amount of time that the pelvis and femoral head maintain contact with each other.[7] The contact between the two is essential for normal formation of the hip joint. The major anatomic factors that contribute to dysplasia are the amount of hip joint laxity of the fetus and the magnitude of acetabular dysplasia. Environmentally, the amount of space that the fetus has to grow in utero plays a role. It is extremely rare for a fetus less than 20 weeks of age to have a hip dislocation.[7]

Orthopedics, Seattle Children's Hospital, Seattle Children's OA.9.120 - Orthopedics Administration, 4800 Sand Point Way NE, Seattle, WA 98105, USA
* Corresponding author.
E-mail address: keith.lemay@seattlechildrens.org

Physician Assist Clin 5 (2020) 487–496
https://doi.org/10.1016/j.cpha.2020.06.009
2405-7991/20/© 2020 Elsevier Inc. All rights reserved.

Genetically determined risk factors for DDH include family history[8] and female sex.[8,9] DDH is associated with an increased or decreased incidence depending on the patient's ethnicity. The incidence of DDH in Native Americans is 76.1 cases per 1000 live births, and it is between 24.6 and 40 cases per 1000 live births in the Sámi ethnic group.[9] The incidence of hip instability of Polish Caucasians is 61.7 cases per 1000 live births.[9] DDH incidence in people of African ethnicity is extremely low. For Africans residing in the United States the incidence is 0.4 cases per 1000 live births, and for Africans residing in Africa it is 0.06 cases per 1000 live births.[9]

Breech position, at any point in the pregnancy, is a major risk factor for hip dysplasia.[7,8] The relative risk of DDH in breech presentation is 3.5.[8] Breech positioning places the hip joint in a position that does not allow it to develop appropriately. Hip dysplasia occurs more frequently in the left hip, as this side is typically forced into adduction by the mother's sacrum.[8] First-born pregnancies are associated with DDH.[8] This might be because there are more first-born pregnancies. However, it has also been theorized that the tight abdominal wall of a first pregnancy increases the deforming forces on the fetus.[7] In second and third pregnancies, the abdominal wall musculature stretches, allowing more space for the fetus. Oligohydramnios has been associated with DDH.[7] The presence of amniotic fluid is thought to protect the fetus from pressure and deforming forces and allows the fetus to move more freely. DDH is associated with the intrauterine crowding conditions of metatarsus adductus and torticollis.[10,11]

Developmental dysplasia of the hip encompasses a spectrum of disease whose severity is broadly categorized on the relationship between the femoral head and the pelvis. Key terms used to describe the disease include: reduced, subluxated, dislocated, stable, unstable, or teratologic.[2] A hip that is able to move from a dislocated, subluxated, or reduced position to any other position on physical examination defines an unstable hip. There are five major types of developmental dysplasia of the hip. In the least severe form of the disease, there is a stable ultrasonographic dysplasia. The acetabulum and the femoral head are in contact with each other, but the depth of the acetabulum is shallow and/or the femoral head is mildly uncovered by the acetabulum. The second form of DDH are reduced hips that are unstable. Subluxated or dislocated, reducible hips are the third form. Dislocated, irreducible hips are the forth form. The fifth form, teratologic or syndromic hip, is one that is dislocated while in utero. Teratologic or syndromic hips are not reducible on examination and may be associated with neuromuscular conditions such as seizure disorders, arthrogryposis, myelodysplasia, cerebral palsy, and myelomeningocele.[2] Teratologic hips invariably do not respond to bracing and require operative intervention to obtain a stable reduction.

Because hip dysplasia is so common, the American Academy of Pediatrics (AAP) standard of care is to perform screening physical examinations on all infants.[2] If the patient has a family history of DDH in a first-degree relative or the patient was in breech position at any point of the pregnancy, the AAP recommends obtaining a screening hip ultrasound at 4 to 6 weeks of age.[2]

To perform a screening or follow-up physical examination for hip dysplasia, tranquility of the infant is critical. A calm, soothing atmosphere allows the infant to relax. That means keeping the temperature of the room warm, dimming the lights, speaking softly, moving slowly, ensuring that the examiner's hands are clean and warm, and using the minimum amount of force necessary. The patient needs all of his or her clothing removed, including the diaper, to allow assessment of asymmetry. Before touching the patient, inspect him or her. One is looking for asymmetry of the body. Do things look the same? Does he or she abduct the legs symmetrically? Is 1 leg over to the side and 1 knee pointed to the ceiling? Are there uneven thigh folds? Examine for other deformities associated with hip dysplasia, such as torticollis and metatarsus adductus. Next, have the infant lay in a prone position and inspect his or her spine. Look at the gluteal folds and inspect for sacral dimples. Palpate the patient's spine, to ensure that it is straight. Observe for asymmetry of gluteal and thigh folds. Asymmetry of the thigh folds is not pathognomonic of hip dysplasia, but it should raise one's suspicion for hip dysplasia.

After that, return the infant to a supine position and perform the Galeazzi test. Flex the hips to 90°; flex the knee joints, and inspect the knee levels for a height difference. If there is a leg length discrepancy, it raises a concern for a possible unilateral hip dislocation. The dislocated side will appear shorter. If both hips are dislocated, a Galeazzi test will be negative, as both of the knees will be the same height.

Next, check for symmetry of abduction. Can the legs be abducted symmetrically? If not, it should raise a suspicion for hip dysplasia. In a young infant, the loss of hip abduction is typically minimal to none.[10] Once the infant is around 3 months of age, it becomes the most sensitive test when evaluating for DDH. The loss of hip abduction results from a gradual contracture of the hip adductors in response to a persistent hip dislocation.[12]

Next check hip stability with the Barlow and Ortolani tests. The Barlow test was initially described in 1962.[12] To perform the Barlow test, place the infant's hips in the position used for the Galeazzi examination. The examiner should place his or her thumb on the medial aspect of the thigh with his or her first web space over the knee joint and the middle and ring fingers on the lateral aspect of the thigh touching the greater trochanter. One should attempt to dislocate 1 hip at a time by pushing the femur posteriorly, like a piston. As one pushes posteriorly, the femoral head may be felt as it exits posteriorly. It is important to examine 1 hip at a time. Do not apply excessive force. One should be able to feel hip instability with light touch (Video 1).

The Ortolani test was initially described in an Italian journal in 1936. Ortolani's description of the test was translated to English in 1976.[13] To perform the Ortolani test, place the hip in an adducted position; then gently abduct the hip and gently push the femoral head anteriorly (see Video 1). It is a positive sign when one feels a palpable, and some even call it an audible, clunk as the femoral head moves from a posterior to anterior position and reduces or relocates within the cavity of the acetabulum.[13] As the child ages, it becomes more difficult to reduce or dislocate the hips. Despite this, it is important to still perform Barlow and Ortolani tests. In the authors' experience, there have been children with positive Barlow and Ortolani examinations up to 18 months of age, especially when associated with joint laxity.

Another test that can be performed is called a Klisic test. The purpose of this test is to detect bilateral hip dislocations. To perform the Klisic test, the examiner should take his or her middle fingers and place them over the greater trochanters. The index fingers should be placed on the anterior superior iliac spine. The index fingers and middle fingers should create a line that point toward the umbilicus. If it does not, it may indicate bilateral dislocated hips.

A red flag when examining an infant or child, is when a child is expressing pain. DDH is not thought to be painful. When the infant or child is inconsolable and screaming when touched, has a current or history of fever, upper respiratory symptoms, or a pseudo-paralysis of a leg, it should raise suspicion for trauma or infection. It is important to remember the physical examination is not 100% reliable, and imaging studies should always be obtained if an infant is presenting with concerns of DDH.

It is important to remember, Ultrasound is the imaging modality of choice for hip dysplasia until the femoral heads ossify around 4 to 6 months of age. The normative values for ultrasound change depending on the maturity of the infant. Ultrasound eval-uation of the infant hip was first described by Graf.[14] He described a morphologic assessment of the hip with an alpha angle and a beta angle. The alpha angle measures the depth of the acetabulum. The alpha angle is the angle formed by a line parallel to the ilium and a second line parallel to the acetabular roof (**Fig. 1**). An alpha angle less than 60° in infants older than 12 weeks of age is considered abnormal.[15] Femoral head coverage is another ultrasonographic measurement clinically utilized. It was first described in the literature by Terjesen.[16] The femoral head coverage expresses the percentage of the femoral head contained within the acetabulum. To calculate femoral head coverage, obtain the same image required to measure the alpha angle. Draw a line parallel to the ilium and extend it past the acetabular roof (see **Fig. 1**). Next identify the femoral head and draw a circle around it. Look at the relationship between the femoral head and the line extending past the acetabular roof. The percentage of the femoral located within the acetabulum, or beneath the line, is the femoral head coverage (see **Fig. 1**). At 12 weeks of age, normal femoral head coverage is considered greater than 50%.[15,17]

In addition to static ultrasound images, Harke described an ultrasound technique of obtaining images of the hip joint in motion, or a dynamic ultrasound.[18] The Harke

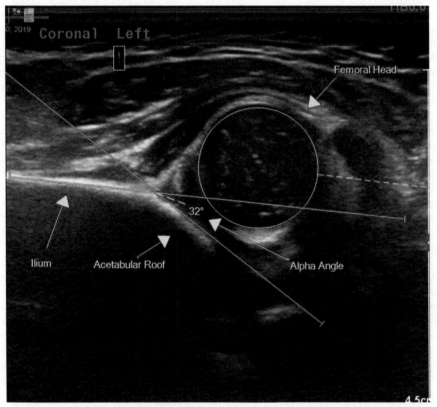

Fig. 1. Hip ultrasound. Alpha angle: Draw a line parallel to the ilium and draw a line parallel to the acetabular roof. The angle between these 2 lines is the alpha angle. Ilium: This is represented by a bright white line. Acetabular roof: This is represented by a bright white line. Femoral head: This is represented by a gray circle.

method assesses for hip stability during the ultrasound examination. It has been criticized for being extremely operator dependent.

Ultrasound interpretation is important when treating DDH. It allows the examiner to not only assess the quality of the image taken but also to assess the accuracy of the measurements reported. In **Fig. 1**, the alpha angle was reported at 47° and the femoral head coverage at 40%. When independent measurements are made, it shows an alpha angle of 32° and a femoral head coverage of approximately 15%.

The ossification of the femoral head around 6 months of age makes it challenging to accurately assess femoral head coverage. It is recommended that after 6 months of age, an anteroposterior (AP) pelvis radiograph be obtained to assess for DDH. It can be challenging to get a true AP pelvis radiograph in an infant. There are several radiographic features to look for when assessing for hip dysplasia. The authors recommend a systematic approach to the pelvis radiograph when evaluating DDH. First, look for the presence of ossification of the femoral heads and for the amount of symmetry between the two. If a femoral head ossific nucleus is not present on radiographs at 6 months of age, do not be overly concerned. In the authors' experience, 40% of infants have femoral head ossification at 4 months of age, 60% at 6 months of age, and 90% at 9 months of age. In addition to lack of femoral head of ossification, the presence of asymmetric femoral head ossification may also be a clue to the presence of hip dysplasia (**Fig. 2**).

Next, measure the acetabular index (**Fig. 3**). This is defined as an angle between a line drawn through the triradiate cartilage (Hilgenreiner's line) and a line drawn through the acetabular roof (see **Fig. 3**). The inferior margin of the iliac bone and the superolateral part of the acetabular roof are used when drawing the line through the acetabular roof. The reference points, particularly in an infant radiograph, are not easy to

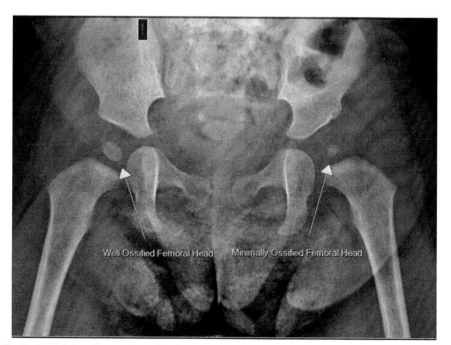

Well Ossified Femoral Head   Minimally Ossified Femoral Head

Fig. 2. AP Pelvis radiograph: In this figure, the right femoral head is well ossified and more developed than the left minimally ossified femoral head.

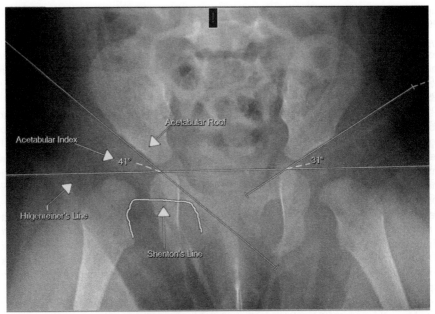

Fig. 3. AP Pelvis radiograph. Hilgenreiner's line is a horizontal line drawn through the triradiate cartilage. Acetabular index is an angular measurement between Hilgenreiner's line and a line drawn through the acetabular roof. Shenton's line is an imaginary line connecting the infero-medial border of the neck of the femur to the inferior aspect of the superior pubic ramus.

determine. Pelvic rotation and pelvic tilt obscure these landmarks. To evaluate for rotation, look at the size of the obturator foramen. If the obturator foramina are asymmetric in size, then the measurement of the acetabular index is less accurate. If the reference points described are not identifiable, the authors recommend using the same reference points between subsequent radiographs to evaluate for change in the acetabular index over time. Measurement of the acetabular index is consistent and reliable, as long as a true AP pelvis radiograph is obtained. The normative values of the acetabular index change as the hip develops. In the authors' experience, at 6 months of age, the upper limit of normal is 30°; at 1 year of age it is 27°, and it is 24° by 24 months of age. This agrees with the findings of Tonnis.[19]

To evaluate Shenton line (see **Fig. 3**), an imaginary line is drawn from the inferior border of the superior pubic ramus along the inferior medial border of the neck of the femur. This line should be smooth and continuous; if not, this could indicate potential hip dysplasia.

To evaluate lateralization, draw Perkin's line perpendicular to Hilgenreiner's line; it should intersect Hilgenreiner's line at the lateral most aspect of the acetabular roof (see **Fig. 3**). The femoral epiphysis should be in the inferior medial quadrant of that line.

When treating DDH, the goal is to obtain and maintain concentric reduction of the hip without significant force. The Pavlik harness is a soft harness with Velcro straps that holds an infant's hips in a flexed and abducted position. This is the ideal position for directing the femoral head toward the triradiate cartilage. The flexion straps prevent extension and hold the hips in flexion, with a goal of 90° to 100° of flexion. The abduction straps prevent hip adduction and hold the hips in abduction. When the hips are maximally adducted together in the harness, the distance between the knees should be no less than 3 finger widths. The harness is worn around the clock, except for bathing until the hips normalize by physical examination and imaging studies. The Pavlik harness only works in a supine position. When infants learn to roll over to a prone position, the harness is ineffective for treating hip dysplasia.

Indications for Pavlik harness treatment include hip instability. Barlow found that 1 of 60 newborn infants are born with unstable hips and that 66% of unstable hips become stable in the first week of life; 88% become stable by 2 months of age without treatment.[12] When an infant less than 4 weeks of age, but greater than 1 week of age comes in with a Barlow-positive hip, the authors start Pavlik harness treatment. Successful treatment for Barlow-positive hips approaches between 94% and 100%.[20] Hips that are Ortolani positive or irreducible require immediate treatment with a Pavlik harness. The Pavlik harness successfully treats Ortolani-positive hips between 64% and 93% of the time and irreducible hips 40% of the time.[20,21] The risk factors for Pavlik harness failure include irreducible hips, bilateral hip dysplasia, and initiating treatment at greater than 7 weeks of age.[22] Treatment for unstable hips may be based on physical examination without ultrasound imaging according to the AAP guidelines.[2]

Pavlik harness treatment should also be used for stable hips that are slow to develop based on ultrasonographic findings. It has been reported that 77% of hips with mild ultrasonographic abnormalities at birth resolved with repeat ultrasound at 4 weeks and 90% at 9 weeks.[23] Thus ultrasounds performed too early (<4 weeks of age) result in several abnormal findings that often resolve on their own. However, waiting too long to perform a screening ultrasound examination wastes valuable time when a patient could be treated with a Pavlik harness. As described previously, the AAP recommends screening between 4 and 6 weeks of age. Because hips develop over time, it is considered reasonable to observe a patient less than 12 weeks of age who has not achieved, but is close to, an alpha angle of 60° and femoral head coverage of 50%. If the infant does not reach an alpha angle of 60° and a femoral head coverage of 50% by 12 weeks of age, then he or she should begin treatment with a Pavlik harness. Children who are being treated for hip dysplasia are left in the harness until they achieve an alpha angle of 60° and head coverage of 50%. The success rate for the Pavlik harness in treating stable hips with ultrasonographic dysplasia is near 100%.[20,24]

Once Pavlik harness treatment is started, schedule follow-up visits for orthotics, physical examination, and ultrasound imaging weekly. At follow-up, answer any questions that the family has about wearing the harness, and evaluate the harness to ensure that it has an appropriate fit. Subsequent follow-ups depend on the severity of disease. Dislocated and subluxated hips need weekly follow-up, whereas stable hips with mild ultrasonographic dysplasia and documented improvement on ultrasound may follow-up in 1 month. Use clinical judgment when determining the frequency of follow-up.

The major complications of the Pavlik harness are femoral nerve palsy, avascular necrosis (AVN) of the femoral head, and Pavlik harness disease. Femoral nerve palsy occurs at a rate of around 2% with Pavlik harness use. Femoral nerve palsy is thought to be more likely to occur in heavier infants and in infants with irreducible hips.[25] Femoral nerve palsy is more likely to occur if the infant's hips are flexed beyond 100° and typically occurs within the first week 87% of the time.[25] To assess for femoral nerve palsy, check to see if the infant is able to extend the knee joint. There is no documentation in the medical literature of the femoral nerve palsy failing to recover. The nerve palsy typically recovers in 5 days, but it may take up to a month for the femoral nerve to fully recover.[25] If a patient develops a femoral nerve palsy, that patient is more likely to fail treatment with a Pavlik harness.[25] It is appropriate to reinstate Pavlik harness use with reduced hip flexion after the nerve has recovered.

Avascular necrosis of the femoral head is the worst complication of Pavlik harness treatment. It occurs at a rate of 2.5 cases per 1000 patients if treatment begins before 2 months of age. If treatment begins after 2 months of age, AVN occurs at a rate of 109 cases per 1000 patients.[2,26] Avascular necrosis is more likely to occur if the hips are abducted beyond 60°.[27]

Another potential complication is Pavlik harness disease. Wearing the Pavlik harness while the hip is dislocated could, in theory, potentiate the posterolateral acetabular deficiency observed in DDH.[28] This occurs if the hip remains dislocated in the Pavlik for prolonged periods without evidence of improvement on ultrasound. Risk of Pavlik harness disease is a reason why dislocated hips require weekly examinations. If these hips do not reduce after 4 weeks of Pavlik harness treatment, the harness is generally discontinued, and the infant referred to a pediatric orthopedic surgeon.

An alternative treatment for DDH is the use of a fixed abduction brace. For practical purposes, it is generally easier when used in bigger infants (typically 3 months or older) who have failed Pavlik harness treatment. If an infant has a subluxated or dislocated hip that is reducible, a fixed abduction brace may be successful if harness treatment failed. One should always confirm hip reduction with an in brace AP pelvis radiograph.

In conclusion, DDH is a common pediatric condition that results in failure of the hip joint to form properly. Early recognition is critical to the successful treatment of DDH. In the United States, all infants are screened with a physical examination, paying special attention to hip stability and range of motion. Infants in breech position at any point the pregnancy or those with an immediate family history of DDH are screened with ultrasound. The main nonsurgical treatments for hip dysplasia are the Pavlik harness and a fixed abduction brace, such as the Rhino cruiser or Ilfeld braces. It is reasonable to initiate treatment for any unstable hip or any hip that has not met standard imaging criteria by 12 weeks of age. The risks of the Pavlik harness treatment are rare but include AVN, Pavlik harness disease, and femoral nerve palsy. Successful treatment of DDH results in significantly improved hip joint function and decreased risk for early onset arthritis and pain in adulthood. At any point in the treatment of infant hip dysplasia, especially if one has a concern that things are not trending as expected, involvement of a pediatric orthopedic surgeon is recommended.

DISCLOSURE

The authors have nothing to disclose.

SUPPLEMENTARY DATA

Supplementary data related to this article can be found online at https://doi.org/10.1016/j.cpha.2020.06.009.

REFERENCES

1. Guille JT, Pizzutillo PD, Macewen GD. Developmental dysplasia of the hip from birth to six months. J Am Acad Orthop Surg 2000;8(4):232–42.
2. Clinical practice guideline: early detection of developmental dysplasia of the hip. Pediatrics 2000;105(4):896–905.
3. Weinstein SL. Natural history of congenital hip dislocation (CDH) and hip dysplasia. Clin Orthop Relat Res 1987;(225):62–76.

4. Wedge JH, Wasylenko MJ. The natural history of congenital dislocation of the hip. Clin Orthop Relat Res 1978;(137):154–62.
5. Smith WS, Ireton RJ, Coleman CR. Sequelae of experimental dislocation of a weight-bearing ball-and-socket joint in a young growing animal. J Bone Joint Surg 1958;40(5):1121–7.
6. Smith WS, Coleman CR, Olix ML, et al. Etiology of congenital dislocation of the hip. J Bone Joint Surg Am 1963;45(3):491–500.
7. Dunn PM. Perinatal observations on the etiology of congenital dislocation of the hip. Clin Orthop Relat Res 1976;(119):11–22..
8. Ortiz-Neira CL, Paolucci EO, Donnon T. A meta-analysis of common risk factors associated with the diagnosis of developmental dysplasia of the hip in newborns. Eur J Radio 2012;81(3):e344–51.
9. Loder RT, Skopelja EN. The epidemiology and demographics of hip dysplasia. ISRN Orthop 2011;2011:1–46.
10. Kumar S, Macewen G. The incidence of hip dysplasia with metatarsus adductus. J Pediatr Orthop 1982;2(3):335.
11. Heideken JV, Green DW, Burke SW, et al. The relationship between developmental dysplasia of the hip and congenital muscular torticollis. J Pediatr Orthop 2006;26(6):805–8.
12. Barlow TG. Early diagnosis and treatment of congenital dislocation of the hip. J Bone Joint Surg Br 1962;44-B(2):292–301.
13. Ortolani M. The classic. Clin Orthop Relat Res 1976;(119):6–10.
14. Graf R. Classification of hip joint dysplasia by means of sonography. Arch Orthop Trauma Surg 1984;102:248–55.
15. Riad JP, Cundy P, Gent RJ, et al. Longitudinal study of normal hip development by ultrasound. J Pediatr Orthop 2005;25(1):5–9.
16. Terjesen T, Bredland T, Berg V. Ultrasound for hip assessment in the newborn. J Bone Joint Surg Br 1989;71-B(5):767–73.
17. Terjesen T. Ultrasound as the primary imaging method in the diagnosis of hip dysplasia in children aged <2 years. J Pediatr Orthop B 1996;5(2):123–9.
18. Harcke HT. Imaging in congenital dislocation and dysplasia of the hip. Clin Orthop Relat Res 1992;22–28..
19. Tönnis D. Normal values of the hip joint for the evaluation of X-rays in children and adults. Clin Orthop Relat Res 1976;(119):39–47..
20. Lerman JA, Emans JB, Millis MB, et al. Early failure of Pavlik harness treatment for developmental hip dysplasia: clinical and ultrasound predictors. J Pediatr Orthop 2001;21(3):348–53.
21. Swaroop VT, Mubarak SJ. Difficult-to-treat Ortolani-positive hip. J Pediatr Orthop 2009;29(3):224–30.
22. Viere RG, Birch JG, Herring JA, et al. Use of the Pavlik harness in congenital dislocation of the hip. An analysis of failures of treatment. J Bone Joint Surg 1990;72(2):238–44.
23. Marks D, Clegg J, Al-Chalabi A. Routine ultrasound screening for neonatal hip instability. Can it abolish late-presenting congenital dislocation of the hip? J Bone Joint Surg Br 1994;76-B(4):534–8.
24. Sucato DJ, Johnston CE, Birch JG, et al. Outcome of ultrasonographic hip abnormalities in clinically stable hips. J Pediatr Orthop 1999;19(6):754.
25. Murnaghan ML, Browne RH, Sucato DJ, et al. Femoral nerve palsy in Pavlik harness treatment for developmental dysplasia of the hip. J Bone Joint Surg 2011;93(5):493–9.

26. Roof AC, Jinguji TM, White KK. Musculoskeletal screening: developmental dysplasia of the hip. Pediatr Ann 2013;42(11):229–35.
27. Kitoh H, Kawasumi M, Ishiguro N. Predictive factors for unsuccessful treatment of developmental dysplasia of the hip by the Pavlik harness. J Pediatr Orthop 2009; 29(6):552–7.
28. Jones GT, Schoenecker PL, Dias LS. Developmental hip dysplasia potentiated by inappropriate use of the Pavlik harness. J Pediatr Orthop 1992;12(6): 722–6.

Anterior Knee Pain in Adolescents
Expanding Your Differential

Leslie Rodriguez, PA-C

KEYWORDS

• Pediatrics • Adolescents • Anterior knee pain • Orthopedics

KEY POINTS

- Understand how basic knee anatomy and clinical presentation can help define the differential diagnosis of anterior knee pain.
- Expand the differential of anterior knee pain, understanding it can be attributed to multiple causes, with the most common factor being overuse.
- Discuss the management of nontraditional pediatric anterior knee pain, and when it requires further workup including diagnostic, laboratory testing, and referrals to subspecialty teams.

OVERVIEW

Anterior knee pain is a common musculoskeletal problem that affects the adolescent population. The differential diagnosis can be challenging to determine when an injury will require further workup. Helping practitioners to create an organized approach will reduce fear of missing a potentially harmful diagnosis. Also giving an overview of common nontraditional causes of knee pain is the goal of this article.

With the increase of youth competitive sports, the incidence rate of anterior knee pain will continue to rise. It is critical for clinicians to create an organized approach to addressing this chief complaint. Current statistics show kids children play an average of 8 hours of organized sports per week outside of physical education in school. They will miss on average 3 weeks of practice or competition because of pain during a season.[1]

ANATOMY

Understanding the anatomy of the knee joint is the foundation to establishing a proper diagnosis (**Fig. 1**). Anteriorly, there are a few important structures to consider. The quadriceps tendon, a part of the extensor mechanism, attaches to the superior pole

Orthopedics and Sports Medicine, Seattle Children's Hospital, 4800 Sandpoint Way Northeast, Seattle, WA 98105, USA
E-mail address: Leslie.rodriguez@seattlechildrens.org

Physician Assist Clin 5 (2020) 497–510
https://doi.org/10.1016/j.cpha.2020.06.006
2405-7991/20/© 2020 Elsevier Inc. All rights reserved.

physicianassistant.theclinics.com

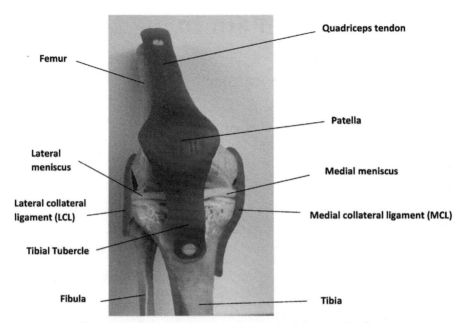

Quadriceps tendon

Femur

Patella

Lateral
meniscus

Medial meniscus

Lateral collateral
ligament (LCL)

Medial collateral ligament (MCL)

Tibial Tubercle

Fibula

Tibia

Fig. 1. Normal knee anatomy using a model, showing both bony and soft tissue structures.

of the patella, and becomes the patellar tendon at the distal pole. The patellar tendon then attaches to the tibial tuberosity on the anterior tibia. These structures play a key role in many traditional causes of anterior knee pain; careful palpation of these structures could reveal the source of pain.

Intra-articularly, the medial and lateral meniscus are located between the femur and tibia. They are the shock absorbers of the knee joint. The cruciate ligaments, both anterior and posterior, provide rotational stability to the knee joint. The collateral ligaments, both medial and lateral, provide additional stability as extra-articular structures from varus and valgus stresses. Reviewing knee anatomy on an anteroposterior (AP) and lateral radiograph (**Fig. 2**A, B) shows the open physes of the proximal tibia, distal femur, proximal fibula, and the closing apophysis of the tibial tubercle. **Fig. 2**C shows a fragmented appearance of the tibial tubercule commonly seen in children with Osgood- Schlatter disease. The patella should be central on the AP view (see **Fig. 2**A) with no signs of patella alta or baja on the lateral view.

HISTORY

History taking is a critical step in collecting information about the patients' anterior knee pain. Asking probing questions, like those mentioned in **Box 1**, will help one navigate the lengthy list of potential causes.

Warmth, swelling, and pain of the knee joint in a child without trauma is much more concerning for infection or inflammatory disorder. Knee pain associated with repetitive stress, increase, or change in training schedule in a growing child is more consistent with apophysitis.[2] Complaints of mechanical symptoms (catching or locking) with reduced range of motion are consistent with an intra-articular injury including a cruciate ligament or meniscus pathology. Feelings of instability could be secondary to patellar instability or quadriceps inhibition.[3] Morning stiffness or pain could indicate an underlying inflammatory condition such as arthritis or chronic recurrent multifocal

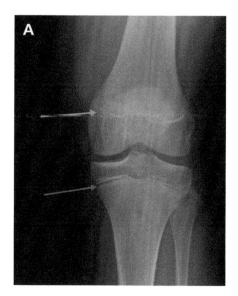
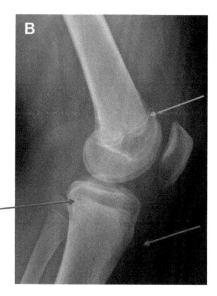
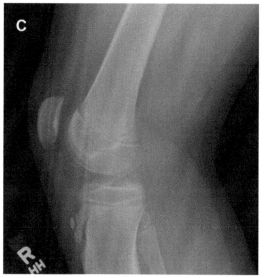

Fig. 2. An AP (*A*) and lateral (*B*) of a normal knee in a skeletally immature child, age 13. Distal femur (*green arrow*) and proximal tibia physes (*blue arrow*) and the tibial tubercle apophysis (*red arrow*) are still open while the child is growing. (*C*) A lateral radiograph shows fragmentation of the tibial tubercule, consistent with Osgood-Schlatter disease.

osteomyelitis. Nighttime pain, with or without systemic symptoms (eg, fever, chills, or night sweats) could suggest a benign or malignant bone tumor such as osteoid osteoma, osteosarcoma, or other systemic malignancies.[4]

PHYSICAL EXAMINATION

Once the history taking is completed, choosing pertinent physical examination tests will further narrow the differential diagnosis. The key for a successful physical

Box 1
Questions asked to determine the cause of anterior knee pain

Question	Concerning Diagnosis
Have you experienced joint swelling?	Infection, inflammatory/rheumatologic, intra-articular injury
Has there been redness or warmth of the knee?	Infection, inflammatory/rheumatologic
Have you experienced any episodes of joint locking?	Intra-articular injury
Have you experienced any giving way episodes?	Intra-articular injury
Do you have joint swelling of any other joints? Ankles? Elbows? Wrists?	Inflammatory/rheumatologic
Did you experience a pop during the time of injury?	Intra-articular injury
Have you had fevers, chills, or night sweats?	Infection, malignancy
Does your pain wake you from sleep? Or is it worse at night time?	Osteoid osteoma, malignancy
Do you experience increased stiffness of the joint when you wake up in the morning?	Inflammatory/rheumatologic

examination lies in understanding the anatomy of the knee joint, along with performing multiple special tests to stress different structures within the knee joint.

INSPECTION

The first step to the physical examination is inspection, assessing for swelling, ecchymosis, or erythema. Swelling is an objective sign the knee joint is irritated, and warrants further investigation. If swelling is present, it is important to distinguish whether it is intra-articular and extra-articular. Extra-articular swelling commonly caused by bursitis tends to be localized and difficult to mobilize. With intra-articular swelling, a fluid wave may be present as the effusion can be milked, and a ballotable patella may be present.[1] Intra-articular joint swelling is not a common finding with typical causes of anterior knee pain such as tendonitis or apophysitis.

Next, watch the patient walk, recording foot progression angle, and monitor for a limp. A normal foot progression angle for an adolescent is 10°, but can range from neutral to 20°.[3] Walking with unilateral increased external rotation could be concerning for a slipped capital femoral epiphysis (SCFE). An SCFE is a diagnosis not to be missed, and can present as diffuse chronic knee pain, with or without a limp.

Measuring the intermalleolar distance will help identify a valgus angular deformity at the knee joint. Although having valgus alignment is not a common cause of knee pain in adolescents, it can predispose a patient to patellar instability, which can cause anterior knee pain. An intermalleolar distance greater than 8 cm after age 7 is concerning for genu valgum that will not resolve, and should be monitored by orthopedic specialist at routine intervals to ensure the problem is not worsening.[5] Although this problem is mainly cosmetic and rarely causes functional impairment, it is important to refer, as a pathologic cause should be ruled out.

RANGE OF MOTION

Range of motion (ROM) is vital to assess; always compare bilaterally, and check both passive and active range of motions. The knee is a hinge joint where normal range is 0° of extension and around 135° of knee flexion.[6] Reduced ROM in knee flexion is common with anterior knee pain, as it stresses the soft tissue structures at the front of the knee. If reduced ROM or pain is present with full extension, it could be anterior fat pad impingement or an intra-articular injury blocking full motion such as a loose body, incarcerated meniscus or ligamentous injury. Intra-articular injuries are more likely to have reductions in both passive and active ROM, with swelling present and sometimes complaints of a locking sensation.

Next, examine surrounding joints, including the hip. An SCFE can present as referred pain to the knee joint. Decreased hip internal rotation, increased unilateral foot progression angle, and pain with hip flexion warrant serious consideration of a possible SCFE diagnosis. Obtain an AP and frog pelvis radiographs. An SCFE diagnosis should warrant immediate attention. The patient should be nonweight bearing on the effected extremity, and an orthopedist should be contacted to discuss likely surgical intervention.

MANUAL MUSCLE TESTING

Manual strength testing can help identify muscle weakness and imbalances. Children who focus on 1 sport and play year round can contribute to development of muscle imbalances (eg, overdeveloped quadriceps muscles in soccer athletes while the hamstrings are underdeveloped).[1] The repetitive nature of sport specialization can lead to overuse injuries, although that topic will not be discussed in detail within this article. Utilizing exercises either under the direction of a physical therapist or through completion of a home exercise program can help eliminate the imbalances. Equalizing muscle development can help reduce the stress on a patellofemoral joint.[4]

The muscle testing should include the quadriceps and hamstrings through resisted knee flexion and extension. Have the patient sit upright, hang his or her legs off the examination table, and flexed at 90°. Evaluate for symmetry and deficiency. Resisted hip flexion, hip abduction, and hip adduction should also be included and be completed with the patient in the same position. An inability to complete a straight leg raise or fully extend the knee while sitting upright, without resistance is known as an extensor lag. The presence of an extensor lag is a sign of weakness in the quadriceps muscle group or injury to the patella or patellar tendon that can be a contributing factor to pain and disability. When referring to physical therapy or a home exercise program, a focus on the vastus medialis oblique (VMO) through isometric contraction exercises can help correct the extensor lag.[3] Improving muscle imbalances can reduce the stresses on the patellofemoral joint, thus resolving anterior knee pain.

FLEXIBILITY

Measure hamstring flexibility through the popliteal angle (**Fig. 3**A), and quadriceps flexibility through Ely test (**Fig. 3**B). Decreased flexibility of both the quadriceps and hamstrings can place increased stress on the patellofemoral joint, which can result in diffuse anterior knee pain.[7] Stressing a dynamic stretching program for youth athletes can reduce pain and help prevent injury in the future.

PALPATION

Identifying the location of the pain and recreating it in clinic can be critical to obtaining the correct diagnosis. Palpate each location separately. Locate the point of maximal tenderness. If a patient has more generalized, diffuse anterior knee pain, it lends to

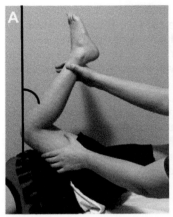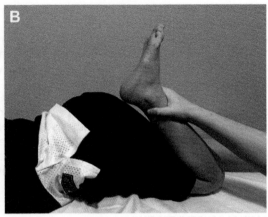

Fig. 3. On the left, (*A*) is the popliteal angle. On the right, (*B*) Ely's test, as shown is positive as the hip has flexed after the knee is flexed.

a diagnosis such as patellofemoral pain syndrome. Pain in a more specific location (eg, the tibial tubercle) would indicate Osgood-Schlatter disease.

Important landmarks to palpate include the distal quadriceps, medial and lateral femoral condyles, patella, medial border of the patella, distal pole of the patella, patellar tendon, Hoffa fat pad, tibial tubercle, and medial and lateral joint line. Tenderness over the medial patella border could indicate a previous patella subluxation/dislocation or medial plica syndrome. Tenderness over the joint line could suggest a meniscus pathology. Pain over the medial or lateral femoral condyles could indicate an osteochondritis dissecans lesion, especially with flexion of the knee joint.

SPECIAL TESTS

There are multiple special tests for the knee joint. Including and understanding different tests will help one expand a differential diagnosis.

Patellar Apprehension

Stressing the patella medially and laterally simulating a subluxation or dislocation will recreate symptoms of apprehension, and worry about the patella dislocating. Ninety percent of patella instability events occur laterally.[3] The patient may reach for the clinician's hands and attempt to stop any lateral movement of the patella in fear of another dislocation. That is positive apprehension. Associated tenderness at the medial patella border where the medial patellofemoral ligament (MPFL) attaches and is commonly injured during a patella dislocation also helps confirm diagnosis.

Ely Test

With the patient prone, passively flex the knee. If the hip simultaneously flexes and lifts off the examination table during knee flexion, the test is positive for quadriceps tightness (see **Fig. 3**B).

Popliteal Angle

With the patient supine, flex the hip and the knee to 90°. Then slowly extend the knee while keeping the hip flexed. Stop when there is increased resistance. Measure the angle, and any angle greater than 50° indicates hamstring tightness (see **Fig. 3**A).

Patellar Grind or Inhibition Test

Placing stress just superior to the patella during isometric quadriceps contraction will create pain and crepitus under the patella. This can indicate potential cartilage damage on the undersurface of the patella.

Collateral Ligament Stress Testing

Stressing the medial collateral ligament (valgus stress) and the lateral collateral (varus stress) with the knee fully extended and flexed at 30° allows assessment of the stability of the ligament. Pain, laxity, and a soft endpoint indicate injury.

McMurray

Axial compression of the knee joint during flexion and extension with internal and external rotation will recreate symptoms. Pain or clunking at the medial or lateral joint line as the knee moves from flexion to extension could indicate a meniscus tear.

Thessaly Test

With the patient standing on the affected leg with it flexed about 30°, rotate with the foot planted from left to right, recreating a plant-and-twist mechanism. A positive test will recreate symptoms of pain over the joint line, and suggest a meniscus tear.

Cruciate Ligament Testing

The Lachmans test and anterior drawer test will stress the anterior cruciate ligament (ACL). The Lachmans test is performed with the patient supine and with slight knee flexion. Stabilize the femur with 1 hand and pull anteriorly on the tibia with the other. The anterior drawer is done with the patient supine and the knee flexed around 90°. Stabilize the foot and pull anteriorly on the tibia. A positive test will show increased ligament laxity with a soft endpoint.

A posterior drawer and sag test will stress the posterior cruciate ligament (PCL). The posterior drawer is done the same as the anterior drawer, but the stress should be posterior rather than anterior on the tibia. A sag test is done with the patient supine and the hip and knee flexed at 90° while holding the foot in the air. If positive, gravity will cause a sagging appearance of the knee.

Wilsons Test

Perform this test while the patient is seated, and knees flexed 90°, hanging off the examination table. Next, have the patient internally rotate the tibia and extend the knee. Repeat this motion with the tibia externally rotated. The patient will feel pain or have crepitus while the examiner palpates the femoral condyle. A positive test could indicate a distal femoral osteochondritis dissecans (OCD) lesion.

DIAGNOSTIC IMAGING

Diagnostic imaging can help distinguish between typical and nontypical knee pain. Plain radiographs are readily available, noninvasive, and relatively low risk to obtain. Weight-bearing AP and lateral are 2 standard views of the knee (see **Fig. 2**). More advanced views include the sunrise or merchant view that allows a better understanding of the patellofemoral joint, and the notch or tunnel view that is helpful to examine the distal femoral condyles.[8]

Radiographs can be helpful to examine osseous abnormalities including cysts, osteochondromas, OCD lesions, or fractures. It can also identify joint effusions and overall joint alignment. Additional radiographs of the surrounding joints, including lumbar, pelvis, or ankle, can also be included if there are concerning signs during physical examination that these joints maybe a potential contributor to the patient's knee pain.

If there is concern for an intra-articular injury, a noncontrast MRI of the knee can provide useful insight to asses for internal derangement. Adding contrast to an MRI can be helpful if there is a concern of malignancy, infection, synovitis, or inflammatory conditions of the joint.[8]

LABORATORY STUDIES

The differential diagnosis of an effusion includes entities previously discussed with intra-articular derangement, joint or systemic inflammatory conditions (ie, juvenile idiopathic arthritis, systemic lupus erythematosus, or inflammatory bowel disease), infection, and nonseptic joint infections (ie, Lyme disease or gonococcal or viral infections).

Bloodwork can be collected from patients suspected of having a septic joint, underlying rheumatological disease, or malignancy. The suspicion will drive the type of laboratory tests obtained. If there is concern for infection, consider ordering a C-reactive protein, erythrocyte sedimentation rate, and complete blood count with differential. If one suspects underlying arthritis or chronic recurring multifocal osteomyelitis (CRMO) rheumatoid factor, antinuclear antibody, HLA-B27, and inflammatory markers CRP and ESR should be considered. If the results show a sign of infection or malignancy, there should be urgent attention to creating a treatment plan.[9]

DIFFERENTIAL DIAGNOSIS

As previously mentioned, the differential diagnosis is long for anterior knee pain. Using the information collected from the physical examination, history and any additional testing it will help narrow the list, leading to a correct diagnosis.

OVERUSE INJURIES

The most common causes of anterior knee pain include overuse injuries that are present in active youth, which include tendinopathies, fat pad impingement, apophysitis (Sinding-Larsen-Johansson syndrome [SLJ] and Osgood Schlatter) and patellofemoral syndrome.[10] These diagnoses are typical causes of anterior knee pain.

History and physical examination will reveal a patient with pain associated with activity and may limit the amount of activity he or she can routinely perform. Rarely, swelling is present, although subjective catching or giving way is not uncommon.

The location of pain is important to help distinguish diagnosis. If over the tibial tubercle, think Osgood Schlatter disease. If the pain is at the distal pole of the patella, think SLJ syndrome. Anterior fat pad impingement causes pain with knee extension and tenderness over the fat pad. Although these diagnoses have similar treatment plans, there is clinical importance to understanding the difference.

INFECTIOUS AND RHEUMATOLOGY

The history taking will reveal a story of likely insidious onset, progressive pain; there could be an association with systemic signs such as fever, chills, or fatigue. On physical examination, one will notice joint swelling, reduced passive, and active range of motion. Joint warmth and erythema are also possible. The patient could be ambulating with an antalgic gait.[11] **Fig. 4** shows a density change within the distal femur, consistent with CRMO.

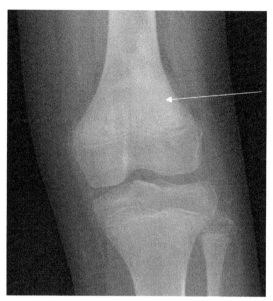

Fig. 4. 12-year-old girl with anterior knee pain. Changes in the density of the distal femur are concerning for infection, in this case chronic recurrent multifocal osteomyelitis. There is bone density changes in the metaphysis of the femur that are consistent with CRMO (cloudy whiteness).

BENIGN BONE TUMORS

Distal femur and proximal tibia osteochondromas are relatively common (**Fig. 5**). They are exposes that extend near the physes and are benign.[12] In general, observation every 6 months with repeat radiographs is sufficient in patients who are asymptomatic. However, some patients present with osteochondromas that grow in size and become problematic with increase in activity. These require surgical referral to discuss resection. It is important to note that many osteochondromas may incidentally found on radiograph and may not be the cause of the patients' knee pain.

Nonossifying fibromas (NOFs) are the most common benign bone tumors in children, and they are generally found incidentally in patients with anterior knee pain. NOFs are benign, will ossify over time and do not cause pain. Observation and reassurance for the patient and family are adequate. The natural evolution of NOFs is to resolve spontaneously within the second or third decade of life (**Fig. 6**).[12]

Nighttime pain that is relieved by nonsteroidal anti-inflammatory drugs (NSAIDs), should raise a red flag for an osteoid osteoma (**Fig. 7**). These benign bone tumors spontaneously resolve over 3 to 5 years. Reassurance and conservative management are acceptable, but if the pain becomes too severe, referral is appropriate. Treatment options include radioablation by interventional radiology, which can resolve symptoms. Advanced imaging with computed tomography (CT) is used to confirm diagnosis and better characterize the lesion.[13]

MALIGNANT BONE TUMORS
Osteosarcoma

Unfortunately, there can be malignant causes for anterior knee pain. Osteosarcomas are most commonly found in the proximal tibia or distal femur (**Fig. 8**). They can

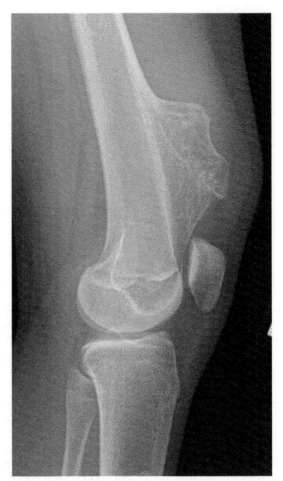

Fig. 5. Large, and likely symptomatic osteochondroma that would require surgical referral to discuss resection.

present as progressive-onset diffuse knee pain and tenderness with concurrent systemic signs.[4] There may or may not be swelling present. This finding requires urgent referral and consultation.

OSTEOCHONDRITIS DISSECANS

A patient presenting with progressive, insidious onset of anterior knee pain with swelling after activity should be concerning for OCD (**Fig. 9**). The most common locations include the distal femoral condyles, although they can also be found on the under surface of the patella.

If an OCD lesion presents on radiograph, refer the patient to orthopedics so further staging of the lesion can be performed. Stable lesions, as determined by advanced imaging (MRI), are commonly treated with activity restriction for 3 to 6 months.[14] This would include low-impact activities including swimming, bike riding, elliptical, and limited running, and jumping. There are multiple stages of OCD lesions; more advanced lesions require operative intervention.

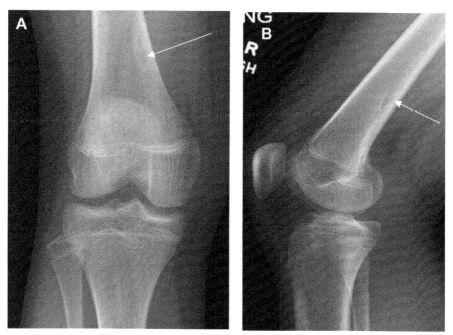

Fig. 6. Small irregularity (*arrows*) at distal medial femur consistent with an NOF. Seen in both the AP (*A*) and lateral (*B*) views of the knee.

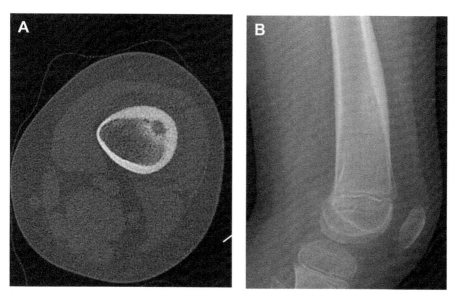

Fig. 7. On the right, a lateral radiograph of the knee (*B*), that shows cortical thickening of the distal femur. The CT on the left (*A*), is an axial cut that shows a nidus, which is a characteristic feature of an osteoid osteoma.

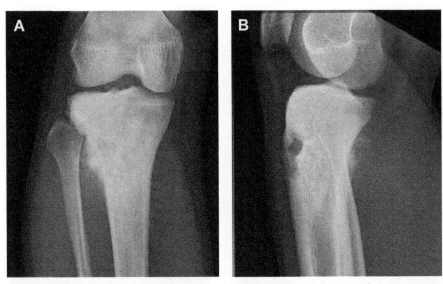

Fig. 8. Aggressive and erosive changes to the proximal tibia consistent with osteosarcoma, seen in both an AP (*A*) and lateral (*B*).

TREATMENT PROTOCOLS

Typical causes of anterior knee pain, as previously discussed, generally improve with activity modifications or restrictions, alternating hot and cold modalities, bracing for comfort, short course anti-inflammatory drugs, and elevation. They may also need temporary protected weight bearing if ambulating is painful. Utilizing physical therapy exercises, with either a home exercise program or formal physical therapy, can address muscle imbalances, improve proprioception and coordination, and address reduced flexibility. Completing 8 to 12 weeks of physical therapy exercises and activity

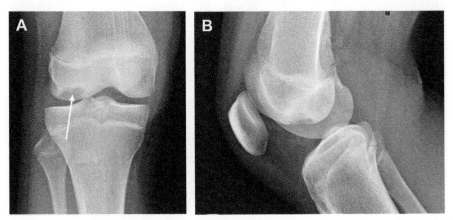

Fig. 9. This is an AP (*A*) and lateral view (*B*) of a 14-year-old boy, with a large osteochondral lesion of the lateral femoral condyle. There is irregularity of the condyle, without obvious loose body or fracture.

restriction will alleviate most typical causes of anterior knee pain.[3] If the patient has persistent pain or evolving symptoms, consider referral to sports medicine or orthopedics for further workup.

Treatment protocols vary greatly depending on the cause behind the anterior knee pain. Beware of nontypical causes of knee pain as discussed in this article. Using clarifying history-taking questions along with confident physical examinations and appropriate radiographs will help a clinician expand his or her differential diagnosis list. Some require referral to an orthopedic specialist and possibly bloodwork, diagnostic imaging, and rehabilitation specialists.

SUMMARY

Adolescent anterior knee pain has a lengthy differential diagnosis list, is commonly secondary to overuse, and will improve with conservative management. Understanding underlying anatomy, asking specific questions about symptoms, and choosing correct physical examination tests will create an organized approach. Always consider uncommon causes of knee pain including SCFE, benign or malignant bone tumors, OCD lesions, infections, or rheumatologic processes during and examination of a patient with knee pain, and utilize available resources to expand the diagnosis list.

DISCLOSURE

The authors have nothing to disclose.

REFERENCES

1. Kodali P, Islam A, Andrish J. Anterior knee pain in the young athlete: diagnosis and treatment. Sports Med Arthrosc Rev 2011;19(1):27–33.
2. Biedert RM, Sanchis-Alfonso V. Sources of anterior knee pain. Clin Sports Med 2002;21(3):335–47.
3. Davids JR. Pediatric knee. Clinical assessment and common disorders. Pediatr Clin North Am 1996;43(5):1067–90.
4. Widhe B, Widhe T. Initial symptoms and clinical features in osteosarcoma and Ewing sarcoma. J Bone Joint Surg Am 2000;82:667–74.
5. Houghton KM. Review for the generalist: evaluation of anterior knee pain. Pediatr Rheumatol 2007;5:8.
6. Shea KG, Pfeiffer R, Curtin M. Idiopathic anterior knee pain in adolescents. Orthop Clin North Am 2003;34(3):377–83.
7. Atanda A, Shah SA, O'Brien K, et al. Osteochondrosis: common cause of pain in growing bones. Am Fam Physician 2011;83(3):285–91.
8. Strouse PJ, Koujok K. Magnetic resonance imaging of the pediatric knee. Top Magn Reson Imaging 2002;13(4):277–94.
9. Ravelli A, Martini A. Juvenile idiopathic arthritis. Lance 2007;369:767–78.
10. LaBella C. Patellofemoral pain syndrome: evaluation and treatment. Prim Care 2004;31(4):977–1003.
11. Kand SN, Sanghere T, Mangwani J, et al. The management of septic arthritis in children: systemic review of the English language literature. J Bone Joint Surg Br 2009;91(9):1127–33.
12. Motamedi K, Seeger LL. Benign bone tumors. Radiol Clin North Am 2011;49: 1115–34.

13. Greenspan A. Benign bone-forming lesions: Osteoma, osteoid osteoma, and osteoblastoma. Clinical, imaging, pathologic, and differential considerations. Skeletal Radiol 1993;22(7):485–500.
14. Madden C, Putukian M, Young C, et al. Knee injuries. In: Maddon C, Putukian M, McCarty E, et al, editors. Netter's sports medicine. Philadelphia: Elsevier; 2010. p. 417–28.

Adolescent Back Pain

Cora Collette Breuner, MD, MPH[a,b,*]

KEYWORDS

- Back pain • Adolescence • Muscle strain • Degenerative disk disease
- Lumbar disk herniation

KEY POINTS

- The prevalence of people of all ages presenting with back pain has steadily increased.
- Recognizing risk factors is essential when conducting the initial interview in an adolescent with back pain.
- A thorough history and physical examination in adolescents with back pain increases early and accurate diagnosis and avoids excessive use of avoidable, costly, or harmful diagnostic tests.

INTRODUCTION

The prevalence of people of all ages presenting with back pain has steadily increased.[1,2] More than 10% of all appointments made by adults with primary care providers are for complaints about back or neck pain.[1] Back pain comprises the fifth most frequent reason for all health care provider visits and costs about $86 billion in health care spending annually.[3,4] Back pain is also increasing in adolescents. One study showed that about 11% of boys and 17% of girls aged 11 to 14 years have experienced moderate or severe low back pain in the past year.[5]

This article observes the World Health Organization definition of adolescents (ages 10–19 years),[6] encompassing early (11–14 years), middle (15–17 years), and part of late (18–21 years) adolescence. Of all adolescent groups combined, an estimated 24% seek medical attention annually for back pain.[5,7] The stage of adolescence is important to be aware of because it changes the predisposition for certain diseases.

Risk factors such as increased childhood obesity, sport specialization during adolescence, and compounding psychosocial and socioeconomic factors also may contribute to the increase in adolescent back pain.[8,9] Back pain can negatively affect quality of life because it correlates with decease in school attendance, poor sleep, and

[a] Department of Pediatrics, Adolescent Medicine Division; [b] Orthopedics and Sports Medicine, Seattle Childrens Hospital, University of Washington, Seattle, WA 98105, USA
* Orthopedics and Sports Medicine, Seattle Childrens Hospital, University of Washington, 4840 Sand point way NE, Suite 200 Seattle, WA 98105.
E-mail address: cora.breuner@seattlechildrens.org

Physician Assist Clin 5 (2020) 511–523
https://doi.org/10.1016/j.cpha.2020.07.001
2405-7991/20/© 2020 Elsevier Inc. All rights reserved.

social isolation.[10] Adolescents with back pain also are more likely to develop chronic back pain as adults.

In a school-based study, a cross-sectional sample of 500 boys (n = 249) and girls (n = 251) aged between 10 and 16 years showed that the average lifetime prevalence of low back pain was 40.2%. Most cases of low back pain were acute episodes that did not lead to disabling consequences. Interestingly, 13.1% experienced recurrent low back pain leading to disabling consequences, with 30.8% experienced loss of physical activity/sports and 26.2% had been absent from school because of low back pain. Recurrent low back pain was particularly evident during late adolescence (20%).[11]

A thorough history and physical examination can increase early detection and accurate diagnosis of low back pain and ensure that costly diagnostic tests are used judiciously (**Table 1**).

Muscle strain is the most common diagnosis among adolescents who present with low back pain. However, clinicians also must be able to recognize more severe musculoskeletal conditions such as scoliosis, spondylolysis, spondylolisthesis, ankylosing spondylitis, degenerative disk disease and herniation, and, rarely, malignancy.

Table 1
Differential diagnosis of back pain in children and adolescents

Presentation	Possible Diagnosis	Associated Symptoms
Nighttime pain	Tumor, infection	Fever, malaise, weight loss
Pain with fever or other generalized symptoms	Tumor, infection	Nighttime pain
Acute pain	Herniated disk, slipped apophysis, spondylolysis Vertebral fracture Muscle strain	Radicular pain, positive straight leg raising test result Other injuries, neurologic loss Muscle tenderness without radiation
Chronic pain	Scheuermann kyphosis Inflammatory spondyloarthropathies Psychological problems	Rigid kyphosis Morning stiffness, sacroiliac joint tender ness —
Pain with spinal forward flexion	Herniated disk, slipped apophysis	Radicular pain, positive straight leg raising test result
Pain with spinal extension	Spondylolysis, spondylolisthesis, lesion or injury in the pedicle or lamina (posterior arch)	Hamstring tightness
Pain with recent-onset scoliosis	Tumor, infection, herniated disk, syrinx Idiopathic scoliosis	Fever, malaise, weight loss, positive straight leg raising test result Symptoms most common in patients 15 years of age and older
Other	Pyelonephritis, sickle cell crisis	Abnormal urinalysis findings, dysuria, fever, other bone pain, history of sickle cell disease

The items in this table are listed by acuteness of symptoms.
From Bernstein RM, Cozen H. Evaluation of back pain in children and adolescents. Am Fam Physician. 2007;76(11):1669–1676.

Importantly, from another study of adolescents (2007–2010) who presented with back pain, tracking them for a year, a total of 215,592 adolescents were identified presenting with low back pain from 2007 to 2010. More than 80% of adolescents with low back pain had no identifiable diagnosis within 1 year.[12]

Although underlying serious disorder is unusual in adolescents with low back pain, clinicians should recognize the specific signs and symptoms that require further evaluation and intervention. Taking a thorough history and performing a concise physical examination guides the initial diagnostic work-up and enhances early detection and accurate diagnosis of adolescents who present with back pain.

ANATOMY AND PHYSIOLOGY

The lumbar spine are common locations for back injury because they bear the weight of the torso and head, as well as cushioning and absorbing pressure during impact (**Fig. 1**).[13]

RISK FACTORS

Recognizing risk factors is essential when conducting the initial interview in an adolescent with back pain:

Family history of low back pain
Concomitant complaints such as night pain, leg numbness, or fevers
Time spent studying in bed or watching television
Posture during computer use
Weight and position of backpack
Height and body mass index[14,15]

Hours, type, and intensity of physical activity: hours and intensity of activity have a bimodal risk for the development of low back pain in adolescents, so weekly physical activity should be quantified. Very active participation in physical activities, defined as

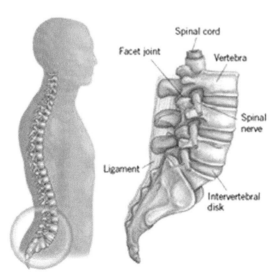

Fig. 1. Spine anatomy. (Reproduced with permission from OrthoInfo. © American Academy of Orthopaedic Surgeons. http://orthoinfo.aaos.org.)

more than 6 h/wk of brisk activity that results in sweating and shortness of breath, is associated with low back pain in male and female adolescents alike.[16] One study reported that back pain has a 1-year prevalence rate of 57% in adolescent athletes compared with 23% in nonathletes of the same age.

Screening Tool

The Keele STarT back screening tool
In the past 2 weeks (yes = 1 point; no = 0 points)[17]:

1. My back pain has spread down my legs at some time in the past 2 weeks
2. I have had pain in the shoulder or neck at some time in the past 2 weeks
3. I have only walked short distances because of my back pain
4. I have dressed more slowly than usual because of back pain
5. I think that it is not really safe for a person with a condition like mine to be physically active
6. Worrying thoughts have been going through my mind a lot of the time
7. I think that my back pain is terrible and it is never going to get any better
8. In general, I have not enjoyed all the things I used to enjoy
9. How bothersome has your back pain been in the past 2 weeks?

Overall: not at all (0 points), slightly (0 points), moderately (0 points), very much (1 point), or extremely (1 point):

- Total of 9 points: 1 point for each "yes" response to questions 1 to 8; question 9 scores 1 point for the responses "very much" or "extremely." The scores are broken down as:
- Less than 3 = low risk; support self-management
- Greater than 4 = medium/high risk; supervised exercise program with or without psychological counseling
- Use subscore from questions 5 to 8 to differentiate medium and high risk
- Less than or equal to 3 = medium risk; supervised exercise program
- Greater than or equal to 4 = high risk; augmented supervised exercise program and psychological counseling

COMMON DIAGNOSES
Muscle Strain

Nonspecific lumbar strain is the most common diagnosis in adolescents with back pain. In a study by Bernstein and Cozen,[18] 24% of adolescents who presented to the emergency department (ED) with low back pain had a muscle strain injury.

Playing sports that involve pushing and pulling heavy weights, such as weightlifting and football, can cause acute lumbar muscle strain.[19] A chronic strain typically occurs after overuse from prolonged, repetitive movements such as rowing or tennis.

Furthermore, adolescents who carry heavy backpacks or who are obese (body mass index >30), which both contribute to poor posture, are at risk for chronic muscle strains. Patients who engage in very limited physical activity, also have a decrease in muscle strength caused by deconditioning, which may predispose to muscle strain.[20]

Clinical examination can guide the next steps in diagnosis. If early identification can be made, associated risks of radiation and further costs of radiology can be removed.[21]

Diagnostic criteria for a muscle strain should include:

Acute, reproducible muscle tenderness

No radiculopathy
Pain related to an injury
Scoliosis

Scoliosis is a lateral curvature of the spine. Not all adolescents with scoliosis experience back pain, but adolescents with idiopathic scoliosis have back pain twice as often as in those without scoliosis, most commonly in the lumbar region.[22] Research shows that, in some cases, genetics plays a role in the development of scoliosis. About 30% of patients with adolescent idiopathic scoliosis have a family history of the condition.[23]

Diagnosing and properly managing back pain in adolescents with idiopathic scoliosis is critically important. Typically, scoliosis is identified during yearly checkups using the Adam forward bend maneuver.[24]

During this maneuver, the patient stands with legs straight and feet together. The patient then bends forward at the waist until the back enters the horizontal plane. The clinician looks for a positive rib hump, which indicates spinal curvature. The accuracy of the Adam forward bend maneuver is impaired in overweight and obese patients because of overlying soft tissue and increased double major (right thoracic and left lumbar) curve presentation. The clinician may need to adjust or include additional physical examination maneuvers, depending on the patient's body habitus.

Spondylolysis and Spondylolisthesis

These diagnoses often manifest with back pain. Criteria for spondylolysis (a bony defect within the pars interarticularis of the vertebral arch and frequent point of fracture) and spondylolisthesis (the forward shift of one vertebra on another) can include:[25,26]

Radiculopathy or neurogenic pain
Intermittent claudication
Difficulty falling asleep or waking up because of pain
Pain worse with sitting and walking
Pain with lumbar spinous process palpation

Adolescent athletes may be at higher risk for development of spondylolysis than nonathletes (13.9% compared with 4.4%, respectively), with gymnastics and weightlifting being the most common causal sports. The history and physical examination is up to 81% specific in patients less than 20 years of age.

Studies have not yet identified physical examination maneuvers that clearly detect spondylolysis; however, a 1-legged hyperextension test is more often positive in patients with spondylolysis.

Although the maneuver cannot be used definitively to justify diagnostic imaging, a positive 1-legged hyperextension test in conjunction with any of the criteria listed earlier should prompt further work-up.

Lumbar spinous process palpation has some usefulness in diagnosing lumbar spondylolisthesis, with a 60% sensitivity and 95% specificity. The diagnosis of spondylolisthesis is difficult because neurogenic and spinal process pain is common in conditions other than spondylolysis and spondylolisthesis.

Ankylosing Spondylitis

This form of arthritis typically affects the spine. Two types affect adolescents: ankylosing spondylitis (in patients aged 17 years and older) and juvenile spondyloarthritis (in those aged 16 years and younger). Both types are more common in men than in women.[27] In 1 study, the presence of 4 out of these 5 criteria showed a sensitivity of 77% and specificity of 91.7% in the diagnosis of spondyloarthitis[28]:

Insidious onset
Patient aged less than 40 years
Pain present at night
Pain improving with exercise
Pain not improving with rest

Other less-specific symptoms that may be present include:

Fatigue
Buttock pain
Morning stiffness
Shortness of breath
Depression

The physical examination should focus on measurement of forward lumbar flexion, lateral lumbar flexion, and chest expansion, because all may be limited in patients with ankylosing spondylitis. Adolescents can have tenderness to palpation of the spine as well as pain in the sacroiliac joints with palpation or stress.[29]

Although not specific to ankylosing spondylitis,[30]: the posterior superior iliac spine distraction test has a sensitivity of 100% and a specificity of 89%, in diagnosing sacroiliac joint dysfunction.

Other concomitant findings may include anterior uveitis, aortic incompetence, cardiac conduction disturbances, and pulmonary fibrosis.[31] Limitations of forward and lateral lumbar flexion may not be as prominent in adolescents with juvenile ankylosing spondylitis compared with those with traditional adult ankylosing spondylitis. Adolescents with juvenile ankylosing spondylitis have shown a greater prevalence of hip disease, including increased circumferential joint space narrowing, osteophytes, erosions, and protrusion acetabulae. With an awareness of juvenile ankylosing spondylitis, health care providers can determine the extent of disease and prevent severe damage.

Degenerative Disk Disease and Lumbar Disk Herniation

Disk-related disorders, including degeneration and herniation, may occur in adolescents with back pain. The term degenerative disk disease can be used to describe a disk with a tear, loss of height, or mild bulging. A disc herniation may develop when one of the intervertebral disks shifts out of position and subsequently pushes on adjacent nerves. Although lumbar disk herniation was found to be less likely (3.5%) in adolescents than most other causes of back pain, it characterizes an important disorder to consider and may progress over time.[32] Health care providers should be aware of risk factors for disk herniation.[33]

Health care providers need to evaluate anthropometrics at each visit because rapid changes in weight or height, or being overweight in general, can put additional stress on the back, making it more susceptible to injury and disk herniation. Adolescent lumbar disk herniation commonly results from sports-related injuries, therefore obtaining a detailed history of activity for patients who participate in high-impact sports or weight-lifting is essential.

In a study by Karademir and colleagues,[33] more than 50% of patients had a family history of lumbar disk herniation, which supports the idea that degenerative disease of the spine may have a genetic predisposition.

Adolescents with lumbar disk herniation can present with radicular pain with or without associated neurologic deficits. Two important neurologic findings to screen for are sensory and motor weakness.

Malignancy

The most common type of bone cancer in adolescent patients is Ewing sarcoma, accounting for 1% of all childhood cancers.[34] Most adolescents with Ewing sarcomas have pain in the area of the tumor. Bone pain can be caused by the tumor spreading under the periosteum, or from a fracture in a bone that has been weakened by the tumor. Patients often have back pain because of the pelvic origin of the tumor. Ewing sarcoma is caused by a gene abnormality of unknown origin, so predictive factors are nearly impossible.[35]

Heath care providers must be suspicious of a malignant process if the patient has low back pain along with night pain, fatigue, fever, and unintentional weight loss.

Ewing sarcomas usually cause a palpable warm lump or swelling, but tumors in the pelvis may not be observed until they have grown large, making physical examination findings nonspecific. Other neurologic signs, such as lower extremity numbness or weakness, loss of coordination of the legs, or loss of bladder or bowel function, often signify that the tumor has already invaded the spinal cord or that the primary cause is a spinal cord tumor, such as a neurofibroma.[36]

Lumbago

This term describes any type of back pain of unknown origin. When a patient does not have a clear cause for back pain, explore other factors, including behavioral health conditions such as anxiety and depression.[37]

Adolescents can be screened for mental health concerns with tools such as the Home, Education and Employment, Activities, Drugs, Sexuality, Suicide/Depression (HEADSS) screening tool, GAD-7 (Generalised Anxiety Disorder Assessment) and PHQ-9 (Patient Health Questionnaire-9).[38]

Establish what has brought the patient to the health care visit. Be aware of the parent and patient's agenda, which may be based on family history, media concerns, or Internet searches.

Socioeconomic status and racial status are associated with significant barriers to access to health care that could prevent long term disabilities and allow all to achieve equitable healthy and productive lives.[39,40]

Genitourinary Tract Disorder

Genitourinary tract diagnoses can cause back pain in adolescents. The history should include questions about dysuria, hematuria, hesitancy, frequency, nocturia, dysmenorrhea, and abdominal pain, as well as diet and hydration status to rule in or out urinary tract infections, kidney stones, and pyelonephritis. Abdominal tenderness, specifically suprapubic, and costovertebral tenderness may be noted in patients with any of the conditions discussed earlier. Vital signs and assessing for hypotension, tachycardia, and fever should be obtained in all adolescent patients presenting with back pain.

Functional Outcomes

Chronic pain in adolescents is defined as persistent or recurring pain for at least 3 months, with a prevalence in the adolescent population of 11% to 38%.[41,42] Pain complaints include abdominal, back, headache, and diffuse musculoskeletal pain (including back pain), which can negatively affect several functional domains, including school attendance and peer relationships, and is associated with comorbid anxiety and/or depression.[43]

Chronic pain syndromes may be challenging for health care providers, patients, and families. Adolescents with chronic pain can become discouraged when others do not believe that their pain exists.

Adolescent perceptions of skepticism by others, including family members, school personnel, peers, and medical providers, can negatively affect self-esteem and psychosocial health. More research is need on this phenomenon.[44,45]

Pain-related stigma has been identified as a public health priority in the 2016 National Pain Strategy,[46] because of its potential impact on delayed diagnosis, treatment bias, delay in diagnosis, and appropriate treatment.

By using the screening tools discussed earlier (HEADSS, GAD-7, PHQ-9), health care providers can help focus the interventions needed to support adolescents with low back pain and decrease stigma, including behavioral health, physical therapy, and integrative therapies such as massage, biofeedback, acupuncture, chiropractic, or a combination therapeutic approach.

Key questions

1. Tell me about how your chronic pain was diagnosed. What was your experience of how doctors initially reacted to your pain?
2. How have teachers and school nurses reacted to your pain? In what ways have they been supportive? In what ways have they not been supportive?
3. Tell me about how other students and friends reacted to your pain? In what ways have they been supportive? In what ways have they not been supportive?
4. How do your parents and/or other members of your family support or do not support your pain condition?
5. Tell me about any time you have felt excluded or treated unfairly by others because of your pain.
6. Tell me about any time you have been made to feel ashamed of your pain.
7. Tell me about any time you have been teased or judged negatively because of your pain.[47]

This topic is included because all health care providers need to be aware of this issue and be comfortable addressing patient and family concerns.

RED FLAGS

The use of a standardized diagnostic algorithm when evaluating adolescents with low back pain ensures that certain red flags are not missed. These red flags are early morning stiffness, gait alterations, irritability or malaise, night pain, numbness, pain lasting more than 4 weeks, muscle rigidity, motor weakness, unintentional weight loss, fever or chills, bowel or bladder changes, and recurrent or worsening pain (**Fig. 2**).

If any of these red flags are discovered, further investigation and more urgent diagnostics are needed, which are described later.[48,49] These diagnostics may be initiated by a primary care provider; however, if neurologic or vascular compromise is of concern, the patient should be seen right away in an ED.

DIAGNOSTIC STUDIES

Various imaging studies can be useful if the patient's history and physical examination provide minimal diagnostic clues. In any adolescent presenting with low back pain, if

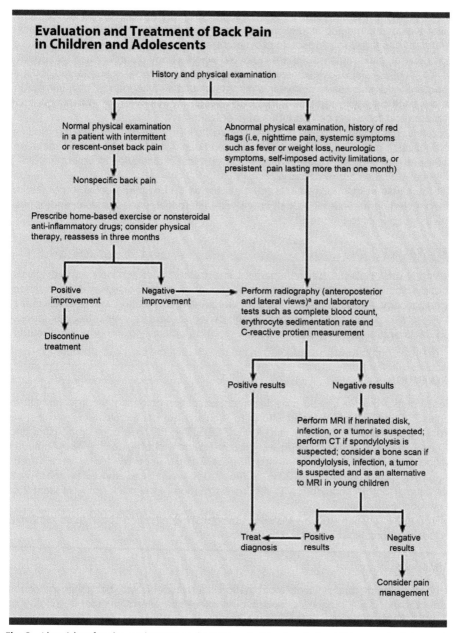

Evaluation and Treatment of Back Pain in Children and Adolescents

History and physical examination

Normal physical examination in a patient with intermittent or rescent-onset back pain

Abnormal physical examination, history of red flags (i.e, nighttime pain, systemic symptoms such as fever or weight loss, neurologic symptoms, self-imposed activity limitations, or presistent pain lasting more than one month)

Nonspecific back pain

Prescribe home-based exercise or nonsteroidal anti-inflammatory drugs; consider physical therapy, reassess in three months

Positive improvement

Negative improvement

Perform radiography (anteroposterior and lateral views)[a] and laboratory tests such as complete blood count, erythrocyte sedimentation rate and C-reactive protien measurement

Discontinue treatment

Positive results

Negative results

Perform MRI if herinated disk, infection, or a tumor is suspected; perform CT if spondylolysis is suspected; consider a bone scan if spondylolysis, infection, a tumor is suspected and as an alternative to MRI in young children

Treat diagnosis

Positive results

Negative results

Consider pain management

Fig. 2. Algorithm for the evaluation and treatment of back pain in children and adolescents. Note: Routine blood work for children younger than 10 years is not included in this algorithm because results can be normal even in patients with leukemia.[41] [a] Oblique radiographs also should be obtained if spondylolysis is suspected. CT, computed tomography. (*From* Feldman DS, Straight JJ, Badra MI, Mohaideen A, Madan SS. Evaluation of an algorithmic approach to pediatric back pain. J Pediatr Orthop. 2006;26(3):353–357; with permission.)

the clinician has no concern for acute fracture and no red flags are identified in the initial evaluation, imaging studies are not recommended until 1 month of conservative treatment has failed to produce improvement.

In general, plain radiographs are indicated when a bony disorder such as spondylolysis, scoliosis, spondylolisthesis, or ankylosing spondylitis is suspected. MRI is appropriate for soft tissue or invasive disorders such as malignancy, disk herniation, or low back pain with radiculopathy. Bone scans are reserved for excluding occult fractures and following certain types of neoplasms.

Clearly, diagnostic imaging is not indicated for every adolescent seeking medical care for back pain. These studies are costly and can result in unnecessary irradiation. Clinicians must rely on a careful history and physical examination to determine when diagnostic studies are necessary.

If the cause of low back pain is not clear based on imaging studies, other testing could include complete blood cell count with differential, urine analysis, and, if indicated, imaging of the kidneys.

REFERRAL

Promptly refer patients for management and treatment of scoliosis, spondylolysis, spondylolisthesis, ankylosing spondylitis, degenerative disk disease and herniation, or malignancy. Although discussing and coordinating any testing with specialists first is the most cost-effective approach, health care providers may elect to order laboratory tests and/or imaging studies before referring patients to orthopedics, rheumatology, or oncology.

PREVENTION

Health care providers should provide patient education on back pain prevention strategies.[50] Providers can support efforts to regularly but not excessively exercise; increase quadriceps, hamstring, and lumbar flexibility; improve core (abdominal and lumbar) strength; and engage in weight management strategies.[51,52] The American Academy of Pediatrics recommends that backpacks used by adolescents should weigh no more than 10% to 20% of their body weight and should be worn with both straps on the shoulders with the lowest portion of the pack riding at least 2 or 3 cm above the waist.[53]

Through education and awareness, appropriate prevention techniques can help reduce the prevalence of back pain in adolescents.[54]

SUMMARY

A thorough history and physical examination in adolescents with back pain increases early and accurate diagnosis, and avoids excessive use of avoidable, costly, or harmful diagnostic tests. Although the most common causes are rarely serious or life threatening, health care providers should be aware of key findings in the history or physical examination that warrant diagnostic imaging or immediate intervention.[55] Health education can reduce the numbers of adolescents with preventable back pain and allow them to lead the happy and healthy life that is their right, and that they deserve.

DISCLOSURE

The author has nothing to disclose.

REFERENCES

1. Mafi JN, McCarthy EP, Davis RB, et al. Worsening trends in the management and treatment of back pain. JAMA Intern Med 2013;173(17):1573–81.
2. MacDonald J, Stuart E, Rodenberg R. Musculoskeletal low back pain in school-aged children: a review. JAMA Pediatr 2017;171(3):280–7.
3. Adar T, Levkovich I, Castel OC, et al. Patient's utilization of primary care: a profile of clinical and administrative reasons for visits in Israel. J Prim Care Community Health 2017;8(4):221–7.
4. Finley CR, Chan DS, Garrison S, et al. What are the most common conditions in primary care? Systematic review. Can Fam Physician 2018;64(11):832–40.
5. Joergensen AC, Hestbaek L, Andersen PK, et al. Epidemiology of spinal pain in children: a study within the Danish National Birth Cohort. Eur J Pediatr 2019;178(5):695–706.
6. World Health Organization. Adolescent health and development. Available at: www.searo.who.int/entity/child_adolescent/topics/adolescent_health/en/. Accessed June 28, 2020.
7. Bhatia NN, Chow G, Timon SJ, et al. Diagnostic modalities for the evaluation of pediatric back pain: a prospective study. J Pediatr Orthop 2008;28(2):230–3.
8. Fett D, Trompeter K, Platen P. Back pain in elite sports: a cross-sectional study on 1114 athletes. PLoS One 2017;12(6):e0180130.
9. Sato T, Ito T, Hirano T, et al. Low back pain in childhood and adolescence: assessment of sports activities. Eur Spine J 2011;20(1):94–9.
10. O'Sullivan PB, Beales DJ, Smith AJ, et al. Low back pain in 17 year olds has substantial impact and represents an important public health disorder: a cross-sectional study. BMC Public Health 2012;12(1):100.
11. Jones MA, Stratton G, Reilly T, et al. A school-based survey of recurrent non-specific low-back pain prevalence and consequences in children. Health Educ Res 2004;19(3):284–9.
12. Yang S, Werner BC, Singla A, et al. Low back pain in adolescents: a 1-year analysis of eventual diagnoses. J Pediatr Orthop 2017;37(5):344–7.
13. Davis E. Lumbar spine anatomy and pain. Available at: www.spine-health.com/conditions/spine-anatomy/lumbar-spine-anatomy-and-pain. Accessed June 28, 2020.
14. Hershkovich O, Friedlander A, Gordon B, et al. Associations of body mass index and body height with low back pain in 829,791 adolescents. Am J Epidemiol 2013;178(4):603–9.
15. Mikkonen PH, Laitinen J, Remes J, et al. Association between overweight and low back pain: a population-based prospective cohort study of adolescents. Spine (Phila Pa 1976) 2013;38(12):1026–33.
16. Auvinen J, Tammelin T, Taimela S, et al. Associations of physical activity and inactivity with low back pain in adolescents. Scand J Med Sci Sports 2008;18(2):188–94.
17. Hill JC, Dunn KM, Lewis M, et al. A primary care back pain screening tool: identifying patient subgroups for initial treatment. Arthritis Rheum 2008;59(5):632–41.
18. Bernstein RM, Cozen H. Evaluation of back pain in children and adolescents. Am Fam Physician 2007;76(11):1669–76.
19. Cleveland Clinic. Back sprains and strains. Available at: https://my.clevelandclinic.org/health/diseases/10265-back-strains-and-sprains. Accessed June 28, 2020.

20. Centers for Disease Control and Prevention. Healthy weight: about child and teen BMI. Available at: www.cdc.gov/healthyweight/assessing/bmi/childrens_bmi/about_childrens_bmi.html#usingBMIcalculator. Accessed June 28, 2020.
21. Alqarni AM, Schneiders AG, Cook CE, et al. Clinical tests to diagnose lumbar spondylolysis and spondylolisthesis: a systematic review. Phys Ther Sport 2015;16(3):268–75.
22. Théroux J, Le May S, Fortin C, et al. Prevalence and management of back pain in adolescent idiopathic scoliosis patients: a retrospective study. Pain Res Manag 2015;20(3):153–7.
23. Menger RP, Sin AH. Adolescent and idiopathic scoliosis. In: StatPearls. Treasure Island (FL): StatPearls Publishing; 2019. p. 1–5.
24. Goodbody CM, Sankar WN, Flynn JM. Presentation of adolescent idiopathic scoliosis: the bigger the kid, the bigger the curve. J Pediatr Orthop 2017;37(1):41–6.
25. Grødahl LH, Fawcett L, Nazareth M, et al. Diagnostic utility of patient history and physical examination data to detect spondylolysis and spondylolisthesis in athletes with low back pain: a systematic review. Man Ther 2016;24:7–17.
26. Sundell CG, Jonsson H, Ådin L, et al. Clinical examination, spondylolysis and adolescent athletes. Int J Sports Med 2013;34(3):263–7.
27. Chen HA, Chen CH, Liao HT, et al. Clinical, functional, and radiographic differences among juvenile-onset, adult-onset, and late-onset ankylosing spondylitis. J Rheumatol 2012;39(5):1013–8.
28. Sieper J, van der Heijde D, Landewé R, et al. New criteria for inflammatory back pain in patients with chronic back pain: a real patient exercise by experts from the Assessment of SpondyloArthritis international Society (ASAS). Ann Rheum Dis 2009;68(6):784–8.
29. Hyphantis T, Kotsis K, Tsifetaki N, et al. The relationship between depressive symptoms, illness perceptions and quality of life in ankylosing spondylitis in comparison to rheumatoid arthritis. Clin Rheumatol 2013;32(5):635–44.
30. Werner CM, Hoch A, Gautier L, et al. Distraction test of the posterior superior iliac spine (PSIS) in the diagnosis of sacroiliac joint arthropathy. BMC Surg 2013;13:52.
31. McVeigh CM, Cairns AP. Diagnosis and management of ankylosing spondylitis. BMJ 2006;333(7568):581–5.
32. Kumar R, Kumar V, Das NK, et al. Adolescent lumbar disc disease: findings and outcome. Childs Nerv Syst 2007;23(11):1295–9.
33. Karademir M, Eser O, Karavelioglu E. Adolescent lumbar disc herniation: impact, diagnosis, and treatment. J Back Musculoskelet Rehabil 2017;30(2):347–52.
34. American Cancer Society. Ewing family of tumors. Available at: www.cancer.org/cancer/ewing-tumor.html. Accessed June 28, 2020.
35. National Institutes of Health. US National Library of Medicine. Genetics Home Reference. Ewing sarcoma. Available at: https://ghr.nlm.nih.gov/condition/ewing-sarcoma#genes. Accessed June 28, 2020.
36. Wilson PE, Oleszek JL, Clayton GH. Pediatric spinal cord tumors and masses. J Spinal Cord Med 2007;30(suppl 1):S15–20.
37. Jonsdottir S, Ahmed H, Tómasson K, et al. Factors associated with chronic and acute back pain in Wales, a cross-sectional study. BMC Musculoskelet Disord 2019;20(1):215.
38. Bright Futures. Performing preventive services: a bright futures handbook. Available at: https://brightfutures.aap.org/Bright%20Futures%20Documents/History,%20Observation,%20and%20Surveillance.pdf. Accessed June 28, 2020.

39. Harper S, Lynch J. Trends in socioeconomic inequalities in adult health behaviors among U.S. states, 1990-2004. Public Health Rep 2007;122(2):177–89.
40. Diderichsen F, Andersen I, Manuel C, et al. Health inequality—determinants and policies. Scand J Public Health 2012;40(8 suppl):12–105.
41. King S, Chambers CT, Huguet A, et al. The epidemiology of chronic pain in children and adolescents revisited: a systematic review. PAIN 2011;152:2729–38.
42. Jordan AL, Eccleston C, Osborn M. Being a parent of the adolescent with complex chronic pain: an interpretative phenomenological analysis. Eur J Pain 2007; 11:49–56.
43. Simons LE, Logan DE, Chastain L, et al. The relation of social functioning to school impairment among adolescents with chronic pain. Clin J Pain 2010;26: 16–22.
44. Forgeron PA, King S, Stinson JN, et al. Social functioning and peer relationships in children and adolescents with chronic pain: a systematic review. Pain Res Manag 2010;15:27–41.
45. Upshur CC, Bacigalupe G, Luckmann R. "They don't want anything to do with you": patient views of primary care management of chronic pain. Pain Med 2010;11:1791–8.
46. NINDS. National pain strategy: a comprehensive population health-level strategy for pain. 2015:1–72. Available at: https://iprcc.nih.gov/sites/default/files/HHSNational_Pain_Strategy_508C.pdf. Accessed June 28, 2020.
47. Wakefield EO, Zempsky WT, Puhl RM, et al. Conceptualizing pain-related stigma in adolescent chronic pain: a literature review and preliminary focus group findings. Pain Rep 2018;3(Suppl 1):e679.
48. Ramirez N, Flynn JM, Hill BW, et al. Evaluation of a systematic approach to pediatric back pain: the utility of magnetic resonance imaging. J Pediatr Orthop 2015; 35(1):28–32.
49. Rodriguez DP, Poussaint TY. Imaging of back pain in children. AJNR Am J Neuroradiol 2010;31(5):787–802.
50. Mettler F. Essentials of radiology. 2nd edition. Philadelphia: Saunders Elsevier; 2005.
51. Taxter AJ, Chauvin NA, Weiss PF. Diagnosis and treatment of low back pain in the pediatric population. Phys Sportsmed 2014;42(1):94–104.
52. Feldman DE, Shrier I, Rossignol M, et al. Risk factors for the development of low back pain in adolescence. Am J Epidemiol 2001;154(1):30–6.
53. American Academy of Pediatrics. Backpack safely. Available at: www.healthychildren.org/English/safety-prevention/at-play/Pages/Backpack-Safety.aspx. Accessed June 28, 2020.
54. Garvick SJ, Creecy C, Miller M, et al. Evaluating low back pain in adolescents. JAAPA 2019;32(12):14–20.
55. Michaleff ZA, Kamper SJ, Maher CG, et al. Low back pain in children and adolescents: a systematic review and meta-analysis evaluating the effectiveness of conservative interventions. Eur Spine J 2014;23:2046–58.

Cerebral Palsy

Etiology, Evaluation, and Management of the Most Common Cause for Pediatric Disability

John Forrest Bennett, MN, ARNP[a],*, Marcella Andrews, PT, MPT[b],
Jaclyn Omura, MD[c,d]

KEYWORDS

- Cerebral palsy • Spasticity • Dystonia • Function

KEY POINTS

- Define cerebral palsy and recognize the proper classification systems.
- Understand pertinent history and physical examination findings in children with cerebral palsy.
- Describe range of tone management treatments including oral medications, injectable medications, intrathecal baclofen pump, and selective dorsal rhizotomy.
- Identify potential musculoskeletal changes in children with cerebral palsy.

INTRODUCTION

Cerebral palsy (CP) is the most common cause of physical disability in childhood. The prevalence is reported to be as high as 3/1000 live births in the United States with 764,000 persons in the United states living with signs of CP.[1] Rates increased toward the end of the twentieth century and have now plateaued.[2] There are a few factors contributing to this trend: increased survival rate among preterm infants, higher incidence of CP reported in term infants, and increased longevity among persons with CP. This population requires specialized care. Early identification allows the care team to offer interventions, such as habilitation and adaptive strategies, that can mitigate the impact of the diagnosis and ensure that individuals with CP reach their maximum functional potential.

[a] Physical Medicine and Rehabilitation, Mary Bridge Children's Hospital, PO Box 5299 MS: 311-1-PMR, 311 South L Street, Tacoma, WA 98415-0299, USA; [b] Seattle Children's Hospital, 4800 Sand Point Way Northeast, Seattle, WA 98105, USA; [c] Rehabilitation Medicine, Seattle Children's Hospital, 4800 Sand Point Way Northeast, Seattle, WA 98105, USA; [d] University of Washington School of Medicine, Seattle, WA, USA
* Corresponding author.
E-mail address: bennettjf@multicare.org

Physician Assist Clin 5 (2020) 525–538
https://doi.org/10.1016/j.cpha.2020.06.004
2405-7991/20/© 2020 Elsevier Inc. All rights reserved.

physicianassistant.theclinics.com

DEFINITION

CP is a heterogeneous clinical syndrome used to describe children who meet specific criteria. CP is defined as "a group of permanent disorders of the development of movement and posture, causing activity limitation that are attributed to non-progressive disturbances that occurred in the developing fetal or infant brain."[3] Key concepts of the clinical syndrome include the following:

- Nonprogressive disturbance: the injury or malformation of the brain is static, and no further injury is expected. Children with metabolic disorders and other progressive disorders do not meet these criteria, whereas they may have clinical features that seem similar to CP.
- Developing brain: the brain injury occurred prenatally, during delivery, or up to 2 years of age. The upper limit of the age range is debated in the literature, and some studies define CP as any brain injury up to 8 years of age.
- Disorder of the development of movement and posture: the child displays motor weakness, poor motor control, hypertonicity, and/or movement disorder.

CP is a clinical diagnosis. Up to 20% of children diagnosed with CP have a normal brain MRI, even though a nonprogressive brain lesion is part of the definition.[4]

RISK FACTORS

There are numerous causes for CP, with some underlying diagnoses difficult to identify. Risk factors for CP are categorized by the period in which brain injury occurs. These periods include prenatal, perinatal, and postnatal.

- Prenatal
  - Infection—can include TORCH (toxoplasmosis, other, rubella, cytomegalovirus, herpes) and chorioamnionitis[5]
  - Maternal complications
  - Multiple gestation
  - Intrauterine growth restriction
- Perinatal
  - Prematurity—this is the number one risk factor for CP. The risk for infants born less than 28 weeks gestation is up to 50 times that of term infants (defined as >37 weeks gestation). Cranial ultrasound findings do not reliably predict diagnosis of CP or classification[6,7]
  - Traumatic delivery—requiring instrumentation or emergency caesarean section[8]
  - Maternal complications—prolonged premature rupture of membranes, placental abruption[9]
  - Seizure
  - Respiratory distress or birth hypoxia
- Postnatal
  - Traumatic brain injury
  - Nonaccidental trauma
  - Hypoxic ischemic encephalopathy
  - Cerebrovascular event
  - Neoplasms

EARLY DETECTION AND DIAGNOSIS

Previously, it was believed that a high-risk infant could not be diagnosed with CP until approximately 12 to 24 months of age, as the practice was to wait and see if motor skills were delayed. This approach is now considered outdated and possibly harmful, as 86% of parents have reported concerns regarding their baby, and a perception that medical information was withheld.[10] With the use of standardized tools at specific times during development, accurate and early diagnosis can be achieved for many babies.

Before 5 months corrected age[10]:

- Neonatal MRI (86%–89% sensitivity)
- Prechtl Qualitative Assessment of General Movements analysis (98% sensitivity)
- Hammersmith Infant Neurologic Examination (HINE) (90% sensitivity)

After 5 months corrected age[10]:

- MRI (86%–89% sensitivity) (where safe and feasible)
- HINE (90% sensitivity)
- Developmental Assessment of Young Children (83% C index)

These tools are best used in combination, which increases the sensitivity. Having an experienced interdisciplinary team trained in the use of these tools, and how to communicate compassionately, is best.

Infants who receive the clinical diagnosis of CP or who are at high risk of CP should be referred for CP-specific interventions. A family concern alone is a valid reason to begin formal diagnostic testing and intervention referrals. Motor cortex activity and development postnatally depends on movement. Without encouragement therapy, the infant is at risk of loss of cortical connections and decreased function. Before starting an intervention, it is helpful to identify the topography (see later discussion), if possible, as the treatments and long-standing outcomes differ.

Current literature supports the following:

- Infants with hemiplegia who receive constraint-induced movement therapy (CIMT) have better hand function[11]
- Infants with bilateral CP with regular hip surveillance have decreased hip displacement[12]
- Infants with any topography who receive Goals-Activity-Motor Enrichment in their home have better motor and cognitive scores at 1 year of age compared with typical treatment[13]

Identifying a child with CP and providing a referral to the appropriate specialist can allow initiation of tone management, therapy referrals, and resultant prevention of musculoskeletal complications. Basic knowledge of CP as well as identification of red flags with a thorough history and physical examination are essential (**Table 1**).

If CP is on the differential diagnosis list, the Quality Standards Subcommittee of the American Academy of Neurology and the Practice Committee of the Child Neurology Society recommend that the diagnosis is confirmed by imaging.[14] The imaging modality of choice is MRI of the brain. Clinically, it is often reasonable to include an MRI of the spine as well to rule out spinal cord injury. Other diagnostic testing to consider includes genetic testing and metabolic disorder workup.

Neuroimaging can confirm the clinical picture and help understand cause of the brain injury. Studies show association between MRI imaging findings and clinical picture.[15]

Table 1
Pertinent findings on history and physical examination to raise suspicion for diagnosis of cerebral palsy in a child

History	Physical Examination
• Presence of risk factors	• Abnormal tone
• Early head control	• Hyperreflexia
○ Because of spasticity in neck extensors	• Persistent primitive reflexes
• Early hand preference (<18 mo)	
○ Seen in hemiplegia	
• Delayed developmental milestones	

- Periventricular leukomalacia: most commonly seen in prematurity, predictive of spastic diplegia but can also be seen in hemiplegia and quadriplegia[15]
- Basal ganglia lesions: predictive of dystonic CP
- Brain malformation: includes polymicrogyria, lissencephaly, and cortical dysplasia, among others. Most commonly associated with hemiplegia, although also associated with triplegia and quadriplegia
- Focal infarcts: most commonly in term infants, predictive of hemiplegia

CLASSIFICATION SYSTEMS

The use of classification systems has emerged as a tactic to characterize an individual's clinical picture and help inform interventions. These include the primary movement disorder, the topographic distribution of impact on the body, and the individual's functional ability.

- Type of movement disorder—there are 4 main motor types described that may emerge and change over the first 2 years. These are spasticity (85%–91%), dyskinesia (4%–7%) including dystonia and athetosis, ataxia (4%–6%), and hypotonia (2%).[14] A physical examination is the best way to identify the type of movement disorder. In some instances, the type of primary movement disorder is unclear. The Hypertonicity Assessment Tool is a valid, reliable discriminative tool that can assist clinicians in identifying movement disorders in CP.[16,17]
- Spasticity—velocity-dependent increase in muscle tone with increased spastic tonic stretch reflex, typically the result of a lesion affecting the pyramidal system. Identification of spasticity requires a thorough neurologic examination, which often reveals other upper motor neuron signs such as hyperreflexia, clonus, and upgoing Babinski reflex.
  - ○ Dystonia—involuntary muscle contractions causing abnormal postures or movements. Can involve the extremities, trunk, tongue, mouth, and eyes.
  - ○ Mixed—both spastic and dystonic, although one can be predominant.
  - ○ Ataxia—difficulty coordinating movements that often results in overshooting/undershooting the target. May affect any part of the body and may lead to problems with speech, swallowing, and coordinating eye movements
  - ○ Hypotonia—decreased tone throughout neck, trunk, and extremities
- Topographic distribution for spasticity—describes the number of extremities affected by the spasticity. Deficits resulting from motor control or weakness are not included when describing the topography of CP, as demonstrated in the case of fine motor impairments in the hands of individuals with spastic diplegia.
  - ○ Monoplegia: one extremity affected

o Diplegia: bilateral lower extremities affected
o Hemiplegia: 1 upper extremity and 1 lower extremity ipsilateral affected
o Triplegia: 3 extremities affected, typically with 2 lowers and 1 upper. The trunk can also be involved.
o Quadriplegia: all 4 extremities affected, the trunk and neck can also be involved
- Gross motor function classification system (GMFCS)—the GMFCS represents the impact CP has on an individual's ability to participate in activities and how much assistance they may require with their gross motor skills.[18] The GMFCS level is described by age, as motor skills evolve and change over time: before 2 years old, 2 to 4 years, 4 to 6 years, 6 to 12 years, and 12 to 18 years.[19] The following text and pictures represent GMFCS levels for children aged 6 to 12 years (when children's motor levels are most stable).
  o Level I—walks without assistive device, can walk up stairs without holding on to railing
  o Level II—walks without assistive device, may get tired over long distances, and need to use railing to go up stairs
  o Level III—requires use of mobility aid to walk short distances and may self-propel a wheelchair over longer distances
  o Level IV—requires use of wheeled mobility device in all settings, may ambulate with assistive device, and hands-on help for therapeutic purposes
  o Level V—dependent use of a manual wheelchair at home and in the community (**Fig. 1**)

A physical therapist can obtain a Gross Motor Function Measure (GMFM-66)[20] to help accurately determine their GMFCS level, which offers predictive data in terms of an individual's functional ability long term, what co-morbid risk factors should be considered, as well as which interventions are most appropriate.[20]

TONE MANAGEMENT STRATEGIES

To date, there is no treatment or cure for the underlying neurologic injury in individuals with CP. However, treatments are offered with the goal of improving function and decreasing the associated complications that occur as a result of the neurologic injury. When treating an individual with CP, it is important to identify the type and severity of motor impairment in order to determine if treatment is necessary. CP affects individuals in many different ways including (**Table 2**):[2]

Clinicians can treat spasticity without significantly affecting an individual's function if they have impaired selective motor control and \ or weakness. When evaluating an individual with CP it is important to include targeted questioning when gathering the history, including the following:

- Sleep

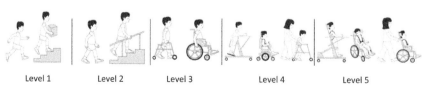

| Level 1 | Level 2 | Level 3 | Level 4 | Level 5 |

Fig. 1. Gross motor function classification system levels. (GMFCS descriptors: Palisano et al. (1997) Dev Med Child Neurol 39:214–23; CanChild: www.canchild.ca. Reprinted with permission.)

Table 2	
Positive and negative upper motor neuron findings	
Positive Upper Motor Neuron Findings	**Negative Upper Motor Neuron Findings**

• Hypertonicity
   Spasticity
   ○ Dystonia
• Clonus
• Hyperreflexia
	• Weakness
	• Impaired selective motor control
	• Impaired sensation
	• Poor coordination

- Feeding
- Function including primary mode of mobility, ability to perform activities of daily living (ADLs), and use of gait aids or equipment
- Pain
- Hypertonicity and its impact on ADLs
- Falls or injuries

A detailed physical examination can quantify and objectively track the deficits of the individual. Physical examination techniques include, but are not limited to, the following:

- Cranial nerve examination
- Deep tendon reflexes
- Assessment of gross motor movements
- Assessment of fine motor control
- Strength testing using manual muscle testing
- Passive range of motion assessment
- Assessment of hypertonicity
- Clinical gait assessment

Performing this detailed examination and history gathering can be difficult within the parameters of today's busy ambulatory clinic setting. The best way to achieve this is to collaborate with an interdisciplinary care team to ensure the best outcome for your patient.

An occupational therapist can use quantitative measures to capture upper extremity function, as well as the Manual Ability Classification System to track and guide upper extremity interventions. A speech therapist can use the Communication Functional Classification System to describe how effective an individual is able to communicate and the Eating and Drinking Ability Classification system to characterize the safety and effectiveness of eating by mouth.[21–23] Many of these measures can be captured and communicated among a care team efficiently providing a clearer clinical picture for each individual and overtime maximize each discipline's impact on an individual's outcome. As these functional measures have evolved, we are transitioning from efficient descriptions of function to objective measures that help guide care.

One powerful assessment tool to achieve this is the ON TRACK assessment.[24] This assessment enables clinicians to score individuals using percentiles within their GMFCS level in multiple categories. ON TRACK compares individuals with their peers and with themselves over time on the categories of strength, range of motion, endurance, balance, health conditions, participation, and self-care. Using these percentiles, the clinician can collaborate with the broader care team to create a targeted plan of care addressing areas of concern, ideally maximizing an individual's function and independence. ON TRACK can be repeated annually and capture the individual's progression based on their GMFCS level.

Treatments of CP are multimodal and include therapies, equipment and bracing, medications, and surgery. A stepwise approach to practice is recommended, and clinicians must understand the interconnected nature of individual treatments. Limited time will be spent on discussing the nuances of different orthotic and therapy approaches given the scope of this article, although one cannot understate the importance that a personalized therapy regimen, appropriate durable medical equipment, and orthotics can play in the functional outcome of individuals with CP (**Fig. 2**).

When focusing on the various medications that are available to treat hypertonicity, one must first determine if the hypertonicity is affecting an individual globally (involving the entire body), or focally (in a select number of muscle groups). Some individuals will have a complex pattern of hypertonicity that affects them focally whereas they additionally have global hypertonicity. The decision to treat hypertonicity and choosing the appropriate medication can be complex. To help guide decision-making it is helpful to understand what tools are available to you as a clinician (**Table 3**).

Surgical interventions and techniques for individuals with CP is evolving. Conceptually there are 2 major types of surgery that target specific deficits that result from CP: orthopedic and neurosurgical.

Orthopedic surgery targets the downstream impacts of hypertonicity, directly addressing the bony and soft tissue ramifications of the neurologic condition. The most common indication for orthopedic surgeries in CP include heel cord contractures, hamstring contractures, hip dysplasia, and scoliosis. Additional orthopedic surgeries can include tendon transfers and upper extremity interventions. The individual's GMFCS level helps identify those who are probable candidates for some of these surgical procedures and can act as a guide to hip surveillance and when to consult an orthopedic surgeon. Improved orthopedic outcomes result from a collaborative approach that includes input and wrap around services from physical therapy and operational therapy, as well as tone management when an individual has hypertonicity.[28]

Neurosurgical options directly target the hypertonicity, a result of CP. **Table 4** summarizes the surgical tone management options.

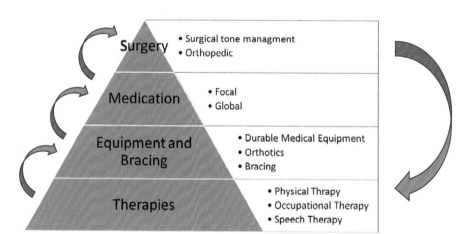

Fig. 2. Management strategies for cerebral palsy.

Table 3
Categorization of medication based on anatomic impact of cerebral palsy[11,25,26]

Focal Hypertonicity	Global Hypertonicity
Onabotulinum toxin A (Botox)	Baclofen
• Affects the presynaptic membrane of the neuromuscular junction, prevents calcium-dependent release of acetylcholine and produces denervation, and persists until new fibrils grow from the nerve and form junction plates on new areas of the muscle-cell walls	• Activates the GABA-B receptors, inhibits transmission of monosynaptic and polysynaptic reflexes in the central nervous system, resulting in relief of muscle spasticity
• Route: intramuscular injections	Diazepam
Phenol 3%–5%	• Binds to receptors on the postsynaptic GABA neuron within the central nervous system enhancing the inhibitory effect of GABA-A receptors. Benzodiazepines do not bind to GABA-B receptors.
• Denatures proteins and causes axonal degeneration	Dantrolene
• Route: intraneural injections	• Acts on skeletal muscle by interfering with release of calcium ion from the sarcoplasmic reticulum
	Tizanidine
	• Central alpha-adrenergic agonist that increases presynaptic inhibition of motor neurons at the alpha-2 adrenergic receptor sites resulting in a reduction in spasticity.
	Dystonia-specific treatment options:[27]
	Trihexyphenidyl
	• Acetylcholine receptor antagonist
	Carbidopa/Levodopa
	• Inhibits peripheral dopamine decarboxylation
	• Serves as a dopamine precursor

Abbreviation: GABA, gamma aminobutyric acid.

MUSCULOSKELETAL DISORDERS IN CEREBRAL PALSY

Scoliosis, hip dysplasia, and other lower extremity disorders are commonly found in individuals with CP. Some individuals also have upper extremity disorders (mostly contractures), although this is less common. Altered skeletal muscle tone associated with CP can interfere with forces across the joints and can lead to contracture over time, as the long bones grow at a faster rate than the skeletal muscle. Poor motor planning, weakness, and truncal hypotonia also contribute to development of musculoskeletal pathology in individuals with CP.

Musculoskeletal pathology in individuals with CP can often lead to pain and deficits in function.[33] Hip and scoliosis surveillance remain an important aspect of care for these patients. **Table 5** will discuss the most common musculoskeletal comorbidities in individuals with CP.

Individuals can present with more than one musculoskeletal system complaint. Contractures and bony deformities are secondary complications of CP and can result in pain and restricted mobility. Single-event multilevel surgery (SEMLS) has become a more widely accepted approach in the last 15 years, as it has been more thoroughly studied. SEMLS aim to correct multiple deformities in one surgery, rather than performing one surgery per year over many years, and can include bony and soft tissue work. Patients and families often report benefit after SEMLS surgery with the research supporting improvements in gait but not necessarily improvement in gross motor function.[38]

Table 4
Comparison of surgical tone management approaches[29-32]

Selective Dorsal Rhizotomy (SDR)	Intrathecal Baclofen (ITB) Therapy

• Surgery on the sensory nerve roots in the spinal canal below the level of the spinal cord
• Neurostimulation used to identify abnormal sensory nerve fibers that are then cut to decrease spasticity and improve motor function
• Patient selection:
  ○ Young child (3–7 y)
  ○ Diagnosis consistent with CP
    ■ Primarily spastic
  ○ Enteral medication maximized without optimal response
  ○ Intensive therapy program without optimal response
  ○ Good strength and motor control
  ○ ROM
  ○ No overt hip dysplasia
  ○ Good follow-through with postoperative care plan from patient/ family anticipated
  ○ Outpatient therapy available
• Potential complications
  ○ Infection
  ○ Spinal fluid leak
  ○ Rare bladder incontinence
  ○ Transient urinary retention
  ○ Rare impotence
  ○ Pain
  ○ Dysesthetic pain
  ○ Incisional pain
	• Nondestructive, adjustable therapy
	• System includes an implantable pump and catheter to deliver precise amount of intrathecal baclofen directly to site of action (GABA receptors) at spinal cord via the cerebrospinal fluid
	• A clinician programmer communicates with the pump via telemetry
	• A fraction of the oral medication dose is needed → minimizes side effects
	• ITB therapy effectively reduces hypertonicity
	• Patient selection
	  ○ Has spasticity or dystonia that is refractory to oral baclofen or have experienced intolerable adverse effects at effective oral doses
	  ○ Sufficient body mass to support pump bulk and weight (usually >15 kg)
	  ○ Social environment conducive to frequent refills (at least every 6 mo)
	  ○ Able to reach ITB provider in case of emergency
	• Potential complications
	  ○ Infection
	  ○ Spinal fluid leak
	  ○ Medication related side effects
	  ○ Baclofen overdose
	    ■ Generalized or rostral progression of hypotonia
	    ■ Drowsiness
	    ■ Lightheadedness
	    ■ Dizziness
	    ■ Somnolence
	    ■ Respiratory depression
	    ■ Seizures
	    ■ Loss of consciousness progressing to coma
	  ○ Baclofen withdrawal
	    ■ Exaggerated rebound spasticity
	    ■ Muscle rigidity
	    ■ Irritability
	    ■ Pruritus
	    ■ Hypotension
	    ■ Paresthesias
	    ■ Fever
	    ■ Altered mental state/hallucinations
	    ■ Rhabdomyolysis (breakdown of skeletal muscle)
	    ■ Multiorgan failure

Table 5
Common musculoskeletal disorders in individuals with cerebral palsy

Joint	Management

Spine
• Scoliosis
  ○ Variable prevalence, 2012 study citing a prevalence rate of 29% in all patients with CP[34]
  ○ Increasing incidence with increasing GMFCS level (IV–V) as well as older age
    ■ Risk of having moderate-to-severe scoliosis at age 18 years is 50% in children of GMFCS level IV–V
  ○ Classically present with long, C-shaped levokyphoscoliosis
	• Not agreed on consensus for surveillance
	• Consider imaging yearly to biannually, depending on patient's GMFCS level and clinical picture[35,36]
	• Imaging modality of choice is XR spine, including posteroanterior and lateral views
	  ○ Degree of scoliosis is measured using Cobb angle, which is measured on posteroanterior radiographs
	• Bracing is not typically recommended for management of neuromuscular scoliosis[36]
	• Surgery considered when curve is approaching 40°, depending on other medical comorbidities

Hip
• Hip dysplasia
  ○ Prevalence of 15%–20% in all patients with CP[37]
    ■ Increased risk with increasing GMFCS level[35]
  ○ Can be a source of pain
  ○ Functional implications include change in gait (if ambulatory), difficulty with seated positioning and hygiene (toileting, diapering)
	• Routine surveillance is recommended, at 12 mo of age.
	• The frequency of imaging dictated by physical examination, GMFCS level, and previous XR findings[12]
	  ○ American Academy for Cerebral Palsy and Developmental Medicine has published a care pathway for hip surveillance
	• Imaging modality includes XR pelvis, anteroposterior view
	  ○ Assess migration percentage that measures the lateral displacement of the femoral head
	• Referral to orthopedic surgeon if migration percentage is >30% of hip abduction <30° on clinical examination

Knee • Patella alta • Patella subluxations/dislocations • Knee flexion contractures	• XR knee 3 views preferred: AP, lateral, and sunrise view ○ Sunrise view particularly helpful for concerns of subluxation/dislocation • Referral to orthopedic surgery for tendon lengthening if knee flexion contractures are limiting function

Ankle
• Equinovarus contractures
  ○ Results from spasticity or dystonia in the plantar flexors and posterior tibialis
  ○ Present with pain, loss of ROM with ankle dorsiflexion
• Ankle valgus, equinus, equinovarus, and planovalgus deformity are also observed
	• Initial management strategies align with tone management strategies discussed earlier, can include stretching, therapy prescription, orthotics, and tone medications
	• Referral to orthopedic surgery for tendon lengthening if contracture is unresponsive to conservative measures or interfering more with functional activities (gait, sitting posture)

OTHER ASSOCIATED CONDITIONS

CP is defined as a disorder of movement and posture, although often individuals with CP can have other medical comorbidities that affect their function and quality of life. A clinician must perform a thorough review of systems to identify comorbidities and offer the proper treatment. A detailed, although not exhaustive, list of common medical comorbidities is listed by system as follows.

- Neurologic
  - Epilepsy: prevalence varies from 15% to 55% in the literature, although increases to around 70% in individuals with CP and moderate-to-severe cognitive impairment.[39] Individuals with hemiplegic and quadriplegic CP are also at higher risk of developing epilepsy
  - Visual impairment (11%): can include retinopathy of prematurity, strabismus, optic neuropathy, and cortical visual impairment
  - Hearing impairment (4%): more commonly seen in individuals with history of kernicterus or hypoxic ischemic encephalopathy as a cause of CP
  - Cognitive impairment: because of the heterogeneous nature of CP, the statistics display variability with a range of 30% to 70%. There is a higher risk in individuals with a concomitant seizure disorder.[40]
- Gastrointestinal
  - Constipation: increasing odds ratio with increasing GMFCS level (IV–V). Because ofdecreased ambulation and mobility, potential medication adverse effects, and slowed gut motility.[41]
  - Gastroesophageal reflux disorder
  - Dysphagia: can necessitate need for gastric tube placement if unable to take in adequate calories to support growth and development
  - Sialorrhea
  - Poor weight gain/malnutrition: Centers for Disease Control and Prevention height and weight growth curves for CP are available to track growth by GMFCS level
- Respiratory
  - Obstructive or central sleep apnea
  - Bronchiectasis: can result from chronic accumulation of secretions
  - Restrictive lung disease: can be seen in patients with moderate-to-severe scoliosis
- Endocrine
  - Puberty occurs within normal age range in most adolescents with CP
  - Metabolic bone disorder: individuals with CP with limited mobility are at high risk of poor bone mineralization and fracture. Vitamin D levels should be checked routinely and supplementation provided when levels are found to be deficient[42]
- Chronic pain
  - Occurs in up to 75% of individuals with CP, related to aberrant biomechanics secondary to motor dysfunction

SUMMARY

CP is the most common cause of pediatric physical disability, which directly affects the health and functional independence of individuals, their families, and their communities. Medical providers should recognize risk factors and physical examination findings that suggest CP. Early diagnosis, collaborative treatment, and evidenced-based interventions can help ensure that individuals with CP reach their maximum potential and quality of life. Routine surveillance for musculoskeletal and other comorbidities is important to provide comprehensive care for individuals with CP. Through targeted use of interventions including CIMT, bracing, therapies, medications, and timed surgical procedures, we can limit the impact of CP on an individual's function and quality of life.

DISCLOSURE

The authors have nothing to disclose.

REFERENCES

1. Christensen D, Van Naarden Braun K, Doernberg NS, et al. Prevalence of cerebral palsy, co-occurring autism spectrum disorders, and motor functioning–Autism and Developmental Disabilities M onitoring N etwork, USA, 2008. Dev Med Child Neurol 2014;56(1):59–65.
2. Graham HK, Thomason P, Novacheck, et al. (2016) Chapter 14: Cerebral palsy.
3. Mutch L, Alberman E, Hagberg B, et al. Cerebral palsy epidemiology: where are we now and where are we going? Dev Med Child Neurol 1992;34(6):547–51.
4. Himmelmann K, Horber V, De La Cruz J, et al. MRI classification system (MRICS) for children with cerebral palsy: development, reliability and recommendations. Dev Med Child Neurol 2017;59(1):57–64.
5. Stegmann BJ, Carey JC. TORCH Infections. Toxoplasmosis, Other (syphilis, varicella-zoster, parvovirus B19), Rubella, Cytomegalovirus (CMV), and Herpes infections. Curr Womens Health Rep 2002;4:253–8.
6. Kuban KC, Allred EN, O'shea TM, et al. Cranial ultrasound lesions in the NICU predict cerebral palsy at age 2 years in children born at extremely low gestational age. J Child Neurol 2009;24(1):63–72.
7. Moster D, Wilcox AJ, Vollset SE, et al. Cerebral palsy among term and postterm births. JAMA 2010;304(9):976–82.
8. McIntyre S, Taitz D, Keogh J, et al. A systematic review of risk factors for cerebral palsy in children born at term in developed countries. Dev Med Child Neurol 2013;55(6):499–508.
9. Accordino F, Consonni S, Fedeli T, et al. Risk factors for cerebral palsy in PPROM and preterm delivery with intact membranes. J Matern Fetal Neonatal Med 2016; 29(23):3854–9.
10. Novak I, Morgan C, Adde L, et al. Early, accurate diagnosis and early intervention in cerebral palsy: advances in diagnosis and treatment. JAMA Pediatr 2017; 171(9):897–907.
11. Novak I, Mcintyre S, Morgan C, et al. A systematic review of interventions for children with Cerebral Palsy: State of the evidence. Dev Med Child Neurol 2013; 55(10):885–910.
12. Wynter M, Gibson N, Kentish M, et al. The consensus statement on hip surveillance for children with Cerebral Palsy: Australian standards of care. J Pediatr Rehabil Med 2011;4(3):183–95.
13. Spittle A, Orton J, Anderson PJ, et al. Early developmental intervention programmes provided post hospital discharge to prevent motor and cognitive impairment in preterm infants. Cochrane Database Syst Rev 2015;(11):CD005495.
14. Ashwal S, Russman BS, Blasco P, et al. Practice Parameter: Diagnostic assessment of the child with cerebral palsy: Report of the Quality Standards

Subcommittee of the American Academy of Neurology and the Practice Committee of the Child Neurology Society. Neurology 2004;62(6):851–63.

15. Bax M, Tydeman C, Flodmark O. Clinical and MRI correlates of cerebral palsy: the European Cerebral Palsy Study. JAMA 2006;296(13):1602–8.

16. Marsico P, Frontzek-Weps V, Balzer J, et al. Hypertonia assessment tool: reliability and validity in children with neuromotor disorders. J Child Neurol 2017;32(1): 132–8.

17. Knights S, Datoo N, Kawamura A, et al. Further evaluation of the scoring, reliability, and validity of the Hypertonia Assessment Tool (HAT). J Child Neurol 2014;29(4):500–4.

18. Palisano R, Rosenbaum P, Walter S, et al. Development and reliability of a system to classify gross motor function in children with cerebral palsy. Dev Med Child Neurol 1997;39(4):214–23.

19. McDowell B. The gross motor function classification system-expanded and revised. Dev Med Child Neurol 2008;50(10):725.

20. Russell DJ, Rosenbaum PL, Cadman DT, et al. The gross motor function measure: a means to evaluate the effects of physical therapy. Deve Med Child Neurol 1989; 31(3):341–52.

21. Eliasson AC, Krumlinde-Sundholm L, Rösblad, et al. The Manual Ability Classification System (MACS) for children with cerebral palsy: scale development and evidence of validity and reliability. Dev Med Child Neurol 2006;48(7):549–54.

22. Hidecker MJC, Paneth N, Rosenbaum PL, et al. Developing and validating the Communication Function Classification System for individuals with cerebral palsy. Dev Med Child Neurol 2011;53(8):704–10.

23. Sellers D, Mandy A, Pennington L, et al. Development and reliability of a system to classify the eating and drinking ability of people with cerebral palsy. Dev Med Child Neurol 2014;56(3):245–51.

24. Bartlett DJ, Gorter JW, Jefferies LM, et al. Longitudinal trajectories and reference centiles for the impact of health conditions on daily activities of children with Cerebral palsy. Dev Med Child Neurol 2019;61:469–476.23.

25. Delgado MR, Hirtz D, Aisen M, et al. Practice parameter: pharmacologic treatment of spasticity in children and adolescents with cerebral palsy (an evidence-based review): report of the Quality Standards Subcommittee of the American Academy of Neurology and the Practice Committee of the Child Neurology Society. Neurology 2010;74(4):336–43.

26. Team, AACPDM Dystonia Care Pathway, D. Fehlings, L. Brown, A. Harvey, K.et al. "DYSTONIA." (2016).

27. Pozin I, Bdolah-Abram T, Ben-Pazi H. Levodopa does not improve function in individuals with dystonic cerebral palsy. J Child Neurol 2013;29(4):534–7.

28. Thomason P, Selber P, Graham HK. Single event multilevel surgery in children with bilateral spastic cerebral palsy: a 5 year prospective cohort study. Gait Posture 2013;37(1):23–8.

29. Bales J, Apkon S, Osorio M, et al. Infra-conus single-level laminectomy for selective dorsal rhizotomy: technical advance. Pediatr Neurosurg 2016;51:284–91.

30. McLaughlin J, Bjornson K, Temkin N, et al. Selective dorsal rhizotomy: meta-analysis of three randomized controlled trials. Dev Med Child Neurol 2002;44:17–25.

31. Park TS, Gaffney PE, Kaufman BA, et al. Selective Lumbosacral dorsal rhizotomy immediately caudal to the conus medullaris for cerebral palsy spasticity. Neurosurgery 1993;33:929–33.

32. Murphy NA, Irwin MCN, Hoff C. Intrathecal baclofen therapy in children with cerebral palsy: Efficacy and complications. Arch Phys Med Rehabil 2002;83(Issue 12):1721–5.
33. Whitney DG, Hurvitz EA, Devlin, et al. Age trajectories of musculoskeletal morbidities in adults with cerebral palsy. Bone 2018;114:285–91.
34. Persson-Bunke M, Hägglund G, Lauge-Pedersen H, et al. Scoliosis in a total population of children with cerebral palsy. Spine 2012;37(12):E708–13.
35. Schroeder KM, Heydemann JA, Beauvais DH. Musculoskeletal Imaging in Cerebral Palsy. Phys Med Rehabil Clin N Am 2019;31(1):39–56.
36. McCarthy JJ, D'Andrea LP, Betz RR, et al. Scoliosis in the child with cerebral palsy. J Am Acad Orthop Surg 2006;14(6):367–75.
37. Hagglund G, Lauge-Pedersen H, Wagner P. Characteristics of children with hip displacement in cerebral palsy. BMC Musculoskelet Disord 2007;8:101.
38. Amirmudin NA, Lavelle G, Theologis T, et al. Multilevel surgery for children with cerebral palsy: a meta-analysis. Pediatrics 2019;143(4):e20183390.
39. Hadjipanayis A, Hadjichristodoulou C, Youroukos S. Epilepsy in patients with cerebral palsy. Dev Med Child Neurol 1997;39(10):659–63.
40. Soo B, Howard JJ, Boyd RN, et al. Hip displacement in cerebral palsy. J Bone Joint Surg Am 2006;88(1):121–9.
41. Veugelers R, Benninga MA, Calis EA, et al. Prevalence and clinical presentation of constipation in children with severe generalized cerebral palsy. Dev Med Child Neurol 2010;52(9):e216–21.
42. Apkon SD, Kecskemethy HH. Bone health in children with cerebral palsy. J Pediatr Rehabil Med 2008;1(2):115–21.

Toeing, Bowing, and Flatfeet in Children

Kids Come in All Shapes and Sizes

Patrick Parenzin, PA-C[a,b,c,*]

KEYWORDS

- In-toeing • Metatarsus adductus • Pes planus • Tibial torsion • Femoral torsion
- Femoral anteversion • Genu varum • Genu valgum

KEY POINTS

- Children's lower extremity shape is dynamic and wide ranging.
- Flat feet are normal and expected in children.
- No shoe, brace, orthotic, or strap will change the shape of a child's bones in the lower extremity.

 Video content accompanies this article at http://www.physicianassistant.theclinics.com.

INTRODUCTION

Kids come in all shapes and sizes. They are a beautiful lot of variability and diversity in what their biologic parents handed down to them through the random combination of DNA. Within the same age group, you can see a variable cornucopia of eye color, hair color, heights, weights, and variation in the shapes of long bones. Much like height and weight are not static in children, a child's lower extremity is ever changing with regard to angular and rotational differences. Understanding what is normal and systematically evaluating a child is key for the clinician caring for pediatric patients.

Chief Complaint: In-Toeing and Flatfeet

In-toeing and flatfeet are daily concerns in the pediatric world of medicine. Each of these concerns carry with them a wide range of normal and abnormal. What is

---

[a] Exercise Physiology, University of Montana, Missoula, MT, USA; [b] Physician Assistant Studies, University of Washington, Seattle, WA, USA; [c] Department of Pediatric Orthopedics, Seattle Children's Hospital, Seattle, WA, USA
* 4800 Sandpoint Way, Seattle, WA 98105, USA.
E-mail address: patrick.parenzin@seattlechildrens.org

Physician Assist Clin 5 (2020) 539–551
https://doi.org/10.1016/j.cpha.2020.06.007
2405-7991/20/© 2020 Elsevier Inc. All rights reserved.

considered normal has a very wide range in children and that normal changes with age. Understanding what is normal requires 3 basic components:

1. Understand the normal progression of rotational and angular variation in a child's lower extremity.
2. A basic physical examination to assess these variations in the lower extremity.
3. By combining 1 and 2, you can distinguish physiologic variants versus pathologic lower limb deformities. Or put simply:

$$1 + 2 = 3.$$

Normal is wide ranging, changes with growth, and requires a certain vernacular to distinguish between physiologic and pathologic. "Version" is the normal twist of the bone and "torsion" is the twist of the bone beyond 2 standard deviations. Torsion is not a bad word and refers to the near end of normal. This being the case, we often use these 2 terms interchangeably.

Metatarsus adductus, tibial torsion, and femoral anteversion are the most common causes of in-toeing and are typically normal findings in children. These normal, physiologic causes of in-toeing originate from the foot, lower leg, or hip, respectively. The pathologic extremes of these are beyond the scope of this article, but we need not be encyclopedias of genetic disorders with lower extremity involvement to recognize what is abnormal. Much like the banker studying a real $100 bill, not a counterfeit, we too can study what is normal and physiologic and in doing so can determine what is pathologic and require further investigation.

STEP 1: THE HISTORY

Like any good patient interaction, a thorough history can often highlight a typical developing child. Who is concerned? Is it grandmother, father, or neighbor? This information is important, because understanding who is concerned will start us down a road toward framing our visit. For instance, if the grandmother is from a culture that puts children in braces and shoes for various pediatric orthopedic concerns, and indeed had 3 of her own children in lower extremity bracing for years, we have a good idea what grandma's expectations are. What is the concern? I like to ask them to point to the body part they are concerned about because, shockingly, "toes pointing in" can mean different things to different people. When does it occur and how long does it last? This question attempts to get at the transient or static nature of the complaint. Is it getting worse or better? Again, we are trying to parse out if the chief complaint is something that is static or if there has been a regression in the child's function. Other basic questions that are key: Does your child have a developmental delay? Did it start suddenly or gradually? Is there a family history of the issue? Is it painful? All of these questions, and many more, attempt to expose an issue that sits outside the normal growth and development of a child.

STEP 2: ASSESSMENT = ROTATIONAL PROFILE

The rotational profile, originally created by Dr Lynn Staheli, is a quick and easy way to assess a child's lower extremity. Composed of 4 basic components, it quickly illuminates physiologic or pathologic lower extremity variations (**Fig. 1**).

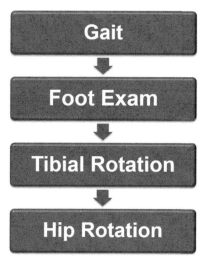

Fig. 1. The rotational profile.

ROTATIONAL PROFILE: GAIT

I start almost every physical examination in the hallway if the child is able to walk (Video 1). This strategy gives them room to run, explore, and hopefully imparts a sense of freedom that is not typically found trapped in an examination room. Roaming the halls with a 2-year-old and their parent you are able to view them from the front and from behind. Does the child limp? Is there symmetry in their gait? Toe-walking? Which way do their feet point? In? Out? This is called their foot progression angle and if the foot points in this is a negative value (**Fig. 2**). If the foot points out this is a positive value.

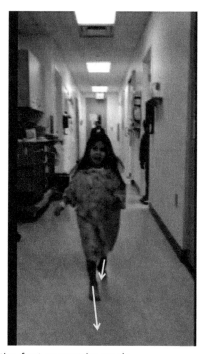

Fig. 2. In-toeing = negative foot progressive angle.

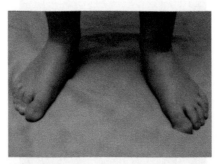

Fig. 3. A child standing with a flatfoot.

If at all possible, always have the child run. Again, this can be fun for many and gives you the chance to unleash your goofy side and wildly run down the hall. This can also shine a bright light on the child that may have a subtle hemiplegia, or other neurologic issue, because running will increase tone. Increased tone will affect their running and — voila! — you just recognized a neurologic problem (and should subsequently complete a thorough neurologic examination so as to not miss something much bigger).

ROTATIONAL PROFILE: FOOT EXAMINATION

Once back in the examination room, observe the child standing. Look at the lateral border of the feet. They should be relatively straight. Do they have an arch? Under the age of 6, most children will have an arch that collapses[1] (**Fig. 3**). Are the arches symmetric? Asymmetry can be a sign of a neurologic issue. Have them go up on their toes. Look to see that their arch gets bigger and their hindfoot drops into varus (**Fig. 4**). Look at the foot while the child is not weight-bearing. They should have a notable arch no matter how flat their foot was in weight bearing (**Fig. 5**). Evaluate the flexibility of the gastrocnemius and soleus by checking dorsiflexion with the knee straight (gastroc) and the knee bent (soleus), respectively (**Fig. 6**). Dorsiflexion should be at or above 20° with the knee straight and above 30° with the knee bent.

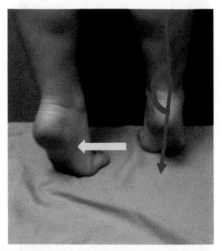

Fig. 4. In a flexible flatfoot, the arch will accentuate on their toes (*yellow arrow*) and the heel drops into varus (*red angle*).

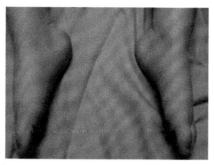

Fig. 5. The nonbearing foot with a notable arch.

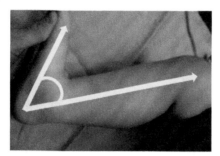

Fig. 6. Dorsiflexing the foot with knee bent and straight test the flexibility of the heel cord.

The Flexible Flatfoot

A foot is not static and the examination must take into account the relationship of the bones and their movement through multiple joints. As outlined, while in standing the foot may indeed have a collapsed longitudinal arch but having the child go up on their toes and observing the foot non-weight-bearing we will see the dynamic shape of a flexible flat foot come to life as the arch appears (See **Fig. 4**).

Most children will develop an arch over their first decade of life.[1] The flexible flatfoot is present in nearly all 2-year-olds and in nearly one-quarter of the adult population.[1,2] Yet as long as the foot remains flexible there are no data to suggest that a flatfoot in an adult is in anyway correlated with pain or disability.[3] So, in essence, because a flexible flatfoot does not cause pain or disability in the child or adult there is no reason to afflict the child with braces, inserts, or rigid orthotics.[4–6] Why attempt to change normal? Yet many feign science and attempt to change a foot's shape with inserts, "special shoes" or rigid devices. These attempts have proven fruitless, as Wenger and colleagues[7] described in their prospective, randomized study of normal children. They demonstrated no treatment effect for shoe modifications and inserts on the development of the longitudinal arch over a 5-year period compared with controls.[7] Again, we see that genetics play a role here; pes planus is often familial (**Fig. 7**).

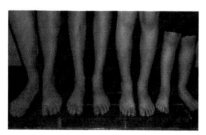

Fig. 7. A family with flat feet. From left to right: 37-year-old mother, 9-year-old boy, 7-year-old boy, and 3-year-old boy.

ROTATIONAL PROFILE: FOOT EXAMINATION, CONTINUED

Looking at the bottom of the foot, draw the heel bisector line (**Fig. 8**). A typical heel bisector line should go through the second and third toe webspace.[8] The more lateral the line, the more adductus is apparent. **Fig. 8** demonstrates metatarsus adductus with a heel bisector line between the fourth and fifth web space. After determining if adductus is present the flexibility of the forefoot should be tested. To do so, hold the heel and direct pressure laterally over the first metatarsal phalangeal joint (yellow arrow **Fig. 9**). The forefoot should go out beyond the lateral foot line (orange line in **Fig. 9**).

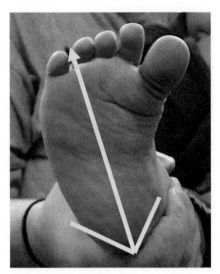

Fig. 8. Heel bisector line in metatarsus adductus.

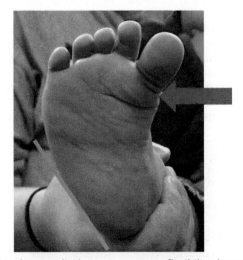

Fig. 9. Lateral foot line (*orange line*). Pressure to test flexibility (*orange arrow*).

Metatarsus Adductus

Metatarsus adductus is the most common cause of in-toeing originating from the foot.[8] Most are flexible and will improve by 12 months of age. Five percent to 10% will be stiff and require casting. Serial casting should be initiated by 6 months of age if rigid.

ROTATIONAL PROFILE: THE TIBIA

Moving the child to the prone position, we will evaluate the shape of the tibia using the thigh–foot angle. Drawing an imaginary line between the foot and thigh we can see if the child's tibia is rotated internally or externally (**Fig. 10**).

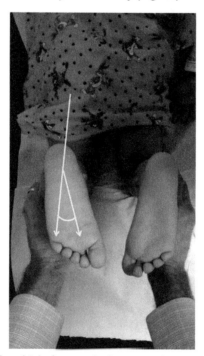

Fig. 10. A 4-year-old with a thigh–foot angle demonstrating internal rotation of the tibia.

Internal Tibial Torsion

Internal tibial torsion (see **Fig 10**) is the most common cause of in-toeing in young children.[9,10] It is common in the 1- to 4-year-old child and can often be asymmetric with the left being greater than the right. The tibia steadily unwinds as the child ages and is typically externally rotated by the age of 6 years. If the child retains the inward spin of the tibia this can lend one to sprinting sports.[11] Again, we see that the shape of the lower extremity is ever changing in a child and retention of the inward spin of the tibia can possibly be a mechanical benefit.

ROTATIONAL PROFILE: ROTATION OF HIP/FEMUR

With the child still in the prone position, we internally (**Fig 11**) and externally rotate the femur.

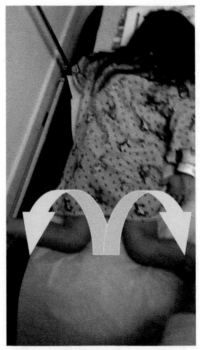

Fig. 11. Internal femoral rotation to 90° in a 4-year-old girl.

Femoral Torsion

Internal rotation of the femur (see **Fig. 11**) is a common cause of in-toeing in children ages 2 to 5.[9,10] It is more common in girls and usually resolves by age 10.[9,10] These are the children that sit in the "W" position (**Fig. 12**) and have an "egg-beater" run. As children age, the femur slowly unwinds but internal rotation can persist in some adults. There is no association with pain, disability, or osteoarthritis if femoral torsion persists into adulthood.[12]

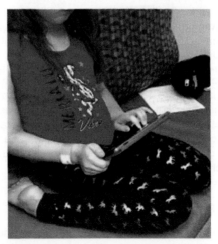

Fig. 12. "W" sitting in the examination room while waiting for the PA to evaluate their in-toeing.

Chief Complaint: Bowed Legs (Genu Varum) or Knock Knees (Genu Valgum)

Angular variations in the lower extremity are common complaints in the pediatric clinic. It is critical to understand that there is a normal progression of angular variation. Most children enter the world with mild genu varum, then slowly develop genu valgum, peaking at 3 to 4 years of age. Genu valgum steadily gives way and is replaced by a straighter profile and by the age of 10 a child has the lower extremities that will carry them into adulthood (**Fig. 13**). This natural progression of angular deformity, although variable by age, is evaluated in the same manner as the rotational complaints. The rotational profile is again used with 1 simple modification: when the child is sitting on the examination room table or in the parent's lap, before moving them into the prone position, simply extend the knees and bring their ankles together for genu varum (**Fig. 14**) or knees together for genu valgum (**Fig. 15**). Measure the distance between the knees (see **Fig. 14**; the intercondylar distance) or ankles (see **Fig. 15**, the intermalleolar distance), respectively.

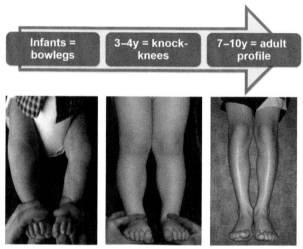

Fig. 13. Normal progression of angular variation in the same child as a newborn (*left*), 3-year-old (*middle*) and 10-year-old (*right*).

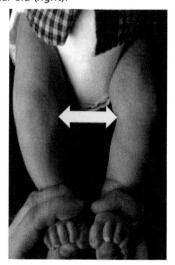

Fig. 14. Genu varum. Intercondylar distance (*yellow arrow*).

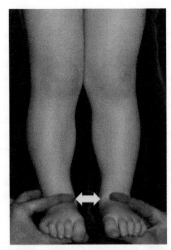

Fig. 15. Genu valgum. Intermalleolar distance (*yellow arrow*).

GENU VARUM

At birth, genu varum should originate from the mid to distal tibia (see **Fig. 14**). This is primarily a "packaging issue" and resolves over the first 2 years of life. When evaluating, measure the intercondylar distance at the knees (see **Fig. 14**, yellow arrow). If the genu varum persists beyond 2 years of age and/or the intercondylar distance exceeds 7 cm the child should be referred to a pediatric orthopedic specialist. Persisting genu varum or excessive intercondylar distance can be the result of pathologic bowing from Blounts disease (**Fig. 16**), Ricketts, skeletal dysplasia, or neurofibromatosis.

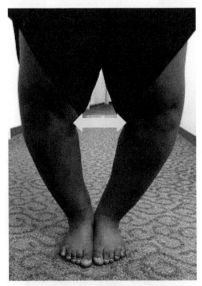

Fig. 16. Blount's disease in a 15-year-old boy resulting in pathologic genu varum.

GENU VALGUM

As a child's tibia slowly looses its varus shape, the medial aspect of the femur and tibia overgrow, resulting in knock knees/genu valgum for most every toddler out there. The peak of genu valgum is at 3 to 4 years of age (see **Fig. 15**). Measure the transmaleolar distance (see **Fig. 15**, yellow arrow). Refer transmaleolar distance greater than 8 to 10 cm or if asymmetry is noted as found after trauma (**Fig. 17**). After 3 to 4 years of age, genu valgum slowly resolves and by 10 years of age most children have their adult profile (see **Fig. 13**).

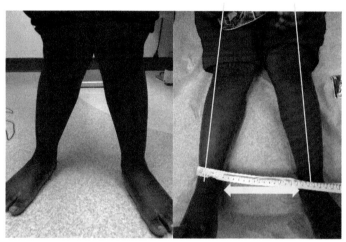

Fig. 17. Unilateral valgus deformity of after an R proximal tibia fracture. Notice the significant transmalleolar distance of 13 to 14 cm.

SUMMARY

The vast majority of rotational and angular deformities are variations of normal, are benign, and resolve with time. Use a thorough history and examination to identify the physiologic normal from the pathologic. Look for normal growth and development and pain or limp with activity. Use the rotational profile to help diagnose the location of the deformity and further evaluate asymmetry if found.

In-toeing, is normal in children and can usually be found in the foot (metatarsus adductus), the tibia (tibial torsion), or the femur (femoral torsion). As the child matures the foot, tibia, and femur slowly unwind and by 10 to 11 years of age a child will have their adult rotational profile. In some instances, in-toeing can persist but is of no concern as long as function is unaffected.

A flexible flatfoot is a normal finding in all toddlers and in nearly one-quarter of the adult population. The longitudinal arch changes over the first decade of life and in most instances is asymptomatic and functional. There is no external force or contraption that need be applied to a normal flexible flat foot as normal will not benefit from treatment.

Angular variations in children are also normal and change with age. Infants begin life with mild genu varum, progress to genu valgum, and then, by 10 years of age, have the lower extremity shape that will carry them into adulthood.

In the instance of every intoeing, flatfoot, genu valgum, and genu varum referral, I give the families a handout written by Dr Lynn Staheli and Dr Vince Mosca titled, "What Parents Should Know About Flatfeet, Intoeing, Bent Legs and Shoes for Children"[13] (**Fig 18**). This handout uses simple illustrations and language to review the material I have just discussed with the family. It is free to download and available in multiple languages thanks to Dr Staheli's Global Help organization. Normal can be a difficult thing to explain, but using the tools acquired as described in this article, I have every confidence that you will be able to convince worried families their child will run, jump, and play no matter which way their foot happens to be pointing.

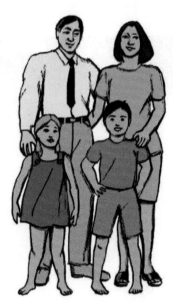

Fig. 18. "What Parents Should Know About Flatfeet, Intoeing, Bent Legs, and Shoes for Children" is a handout created by Dr Lynn Staheli and Dr Vince Mosca. It is available in multiple languages and formats and provides information for families about common developmental variations in infants and children. It is a free resource and can be found at Dr Staheli's website: global-help.org. (*Courtesy of* Lynn Staheli.)

DISCLOSURE

The author has nothing to disclose.

SUPPLEMENTARY DATA

Supplementary data related to this article can be found online at https://doi.org/10.1016/j.cpha.2020.06.007.

REFERENCES

1. Staheli LT, Chew DE, Corbett M. The longitudinal arch. A survey of eight hundred and eighty-two feet in normal children and adults. J Bone Joint Surg Am 1987;69:426–8.
2. Morley AJ. Knock-knee in children. Br Med J 1957;2:976–9.
3. Carr J II, Yang S, Lather LA. Pediatric pes planus: a state-of-the-art review. Pediatrics 2016;137(3):e20151230.

4. Mosca VS. Flexible flatfoot in children and adolescents. J Child Orthop 2010;4(2): 107–21.
5. Staheli L. Planovalgus foot deformity: current status. J Am Podiatr Med Assoc 1999;89:94–9.
6. Pfeiffer M, Kotz R, Ledl T, et al. Prevalence of flat foot in preschool-aged children. Pediatrics 2006;118(2):634–9.
7. Wenger DR, Mauldin D, Speck G, et al. Corrective shoes and inserts as treatment for flexible flatfoot in infants and children. J Bone Joint Surg Am 1989;71:800–10.
8. Bleck EE. Metatarsus adductus: classification and relationship to outcomes of treatment. J Pediatr Orthop 1983;3(1):2–9.
9. Staheli L, Mosca V. What parents should know about flatfeet, intoeing, bent legs and shoes for children. Seattle: Global-HELP Publication, Staheli, Inc; 1979.
10. Staheli LT. Practice of pediatric orthopedics. Seattle: Lippincott; 2002.
11. Fuchs R, Staheli L. Sprinting and Intoeing. J Pediatr Orthop 1996;16(4):489–91.
12. Kitaoka HB, Weiner DS, Cook AJ, et al. Relationship between femoral anteversion and osteoarthritis of the hip. J Pediatr Orthop 1980;9(4):396–404.
13. Global-Help. Available at: http://www.globalhelp.org/publications/books/book_whatparentsflatfeet.html. Accessed July 17, 2020.

Printed and bound by CPI Group (UK) Ltd, Croydon, CR0 4YY

07/10/2024

01041951-0003